THE EPILEPSY HANDBOOK
The Practical Management of Seizures

Second Edition

The Epilepsy Handbook
The Practical Management of Seizures
Second Edition

Robert J. Gumnit, M.D.

President, MINCEP® Epilepsy Care
Minnesota Comprehensive Epilepsy Program, P.A.
Minneapolis, Minnesota

Clinical Professor of Neurology and Neurosurgery
Director, Epilepsy Clinical Research Program
Department of Neurology
University of Minnesota
Minneapolis, Minnesota

Raven Press  New York

Library of Congress Cataloging-in-Publication Data

Gumnit, Robert J.
    The epilepsy handbook : the practical management of seizures /
Robert J. Gumnit.—2nd ed.
      p. cm.
    Includes bibliographical references and index.
    ISBN 0-7817-0176-7
    1. Epilepsy—Chemotherapy—Handbooks, manuals, etc.
  2. Anticonvulsants—Handbooks, manuals, etc. I. Title.
    [DNLM: 1. Epilepsy—therapy—handbooks.
  2. Convulsions—therapy—handbooks. WL 39 G974e 1994]
  RC374.C48G85 1994
  616.8′53061—dc20
  DNLM/DLC
  for Library of Congress

                                  94-18362
                                      CIP

Contents

Preface

In 1976, the author first edited a "Handbook for Physicians" on behalf of the Minnesota Comprehensive Epilepsy Program. *The Epilepsy Handbook* first appeared in this format in 1983. This second edition has been largely rewritten. The book is written for primary care physicians, but also will be useful to psychologists, nurses, vocational counselors, and others working with the patient with seizures.

Some of the information has been presented in terms less technical than might be expected. This was a deliberate choice in order to make the book more accessible to other health professionals who work with the physician. Psychological, nursing, and vocational information has been presented along with the medical in order to demonstrate how the efforts of various members of the team inter-relate.

I have adopted the practice of using male and female pronouns in alternate chapters throughout the book. His/her is an ugly construction and sentences become unnecessarily complex if one attempts to use only neuter pronouns, the third person, or the indirect voice. Seizures do not discriminate between the sexes, and neither do I.

Acknowledgments

My colleagues at MINCEP® Epilepsy Care (Minnesota Comprehensive Epilepsy Program, P.A.) and the University of Minnesota have made valuable contributions to my understanding of epilepsy and to the development of the book. I am greatly indebted to all of them. I am sure that I have unconsciously used many ideas and words they have given to me. In some instances, I have used material on which we worked together and which previously appeared in various scientific papers and pamphlets.

Introduction

The information presented in this book is as up-to-date as I could make it. The physician should not hesitate to use it as a ready guide, but no book can be guaranteed to be completely accurate.

The opinions and recommendations in this handbook are based on statements in the scientific literature and on the research and personal experience of the author. These recommendations are general guidelines and are not prescriptive. Physicians should consult the recommendations provided by product manufacturers and use their own judgment.

Epilepsy is not a disease, it is a constellation of symptoms. Therefore, there is no "cure" for epilepsy. Some of the causes of epilepsy can be cured. In most cases, even if a cure is not possible, complete control of seizures can be brought about. In nearly all cases, improvement in the quality of life of the patient can be obtained. In common with most chronic diseases, epilepsy requires long-term, continuing concerned treatment with a multispecialty approach.

Early Intervention

Seizures are not good for the brain and disability is not good for the soul. Major interventions are more successful when carried out early. The average patient referred to MINCEP has had seizures for 14 years. We don't let people have gall bladder attacks for 14 years! The modern treatment of epilepsy is as effective as our treatment of gall bladder disease.

A Note About References

The treatment of epilepsy is rapidly changing. If this book is to be useful for more than a brief time, it should emphasize general principles. Therefore, I have chosen to refer to a few key articles or books (when they exist) that can serve as an introduction to the literature and provide additional details. The reader should consult databases such as Medline or the National Epilepsy Library of the Epilepsy Foundation of America for references. In this way, up-to-date publications can be located. Key words for searching include epilepsy, seizures, psychogenic seizures, non-epileptic events, antiepileptic drugs, drug toxicity, and epilepsy surgery.

GENERAL REFERENCES

Aicardi J. *Diseases of the nervous system in childhood.* Chapters 16, 17 and 30. Mac Keith Press, London.

Dam M, Lennart G. *Comprehensive epileptology.* New York: Raven Press, 1991.

Engel Jr, J. *Seizures and epilepsy. contemporary neurology series,* Vol. 31. Philadelphia: F.A. Davis Company, 1989.

Engel, Jerome Jr., ed. *Surgical treatment of the epilepsies.* 2nd ed. New York, Raven Press, 1993.

Gumnit RJ. *Living well with epilepsy.* New York: Demos Press, 1990.

Gumnit RJ. *Help your child live well with epilepsy.* New York: Demos Press, 1994.

Hauser WA, Hesdorffer, DC. *Epilepsy: Frequency, causes and consequences.* New York: Demos Press, 1990.

Hauser WA. *Current trends in epilepsy: A self-study course for physicians.* Landover, Maryland: Epilepsy Foundation of America, 1988.

Gumnit RJ, Leppik IE. The epilepsies. In: Rosenberg, RN, ed. *Comprehensive neurology.* New York: Raven Press, 1991:311–336.

Luders HO. *Epilepsy surgery.* New York: Raven Press, 1992.

Wyllie E. *The treatment of epilepsy: Principles and practice.* Philadelphia: Lea and Febiger, 1993.

Physicians may telephone the National Epilepsy Library at the Epilepsy Foundation of America (1-800-EFA-4050) for help with up-to-date scientific information.

THE EPILEPSY HANDBOOK
The Practical Management of Seizures

Second Edition

<table><tr><td>1</td><td># What Are Seizures? What Is Epilepsy?</td></tr></table>

DEFINITIONS

The term epilepsy, in modern usage, means little more than a condition in which a patient has recurrent seizures. If someone had three seizures during a bout of meningitis, and if the seizures did not recur later, we would not describe the person as having epilepsy. However, if someone had two seizures of unknown cause, occurring six months apart, a diagnosis of epilepsy would be correct.

Many years ago, the word epilepsy had two additional connotations. There was the implication that the disorder was influenced by heredity. This, indeed, is the case in certain instances. (See the section on genetics, Chapter 5.) There was also the concept of an epileptic diathesis, implying that every individual has a threshold for the appearance of seizures and that anyone can have a seizure under appropriate circumstances. This is true, but some people have a higher threshold than others and appear to be more resistant to seizures. This concept is of great importance in treating the patient. It emphasizes that we have to understand both the basic underlying brain status of the individual and the specific factors that might provoke a seizure at any given time.

PREVALENCE AND INCIDENCE

The prevalence and incidence of epilepsy are difficult to establish because of problems with both diagnosis and reporting. Although epilepsy is not a disease, we can define it as a condition in which someone has had at least two seizures at separate times sometime in their life. Therefore, we need information about two categories of people: those who have had a single seizure, and those who have had recurrent seizures and thus can be diagnosed as having epilepsy.

The best information on the incidence and prevalence of epilepsy has come from Olmstead County, Minnesota, a predominantly white, middle class, agricultural community. Studies have shown that 9% of that population (1 out of every 11 people) have experienced a seizure sometime in their life. Although 2% to 3% have experienced only simple febrile seizures, 3% have experienced recurrent seizures, thus meeting the criteria for the diagnosis of epilepsy. An additional 3% have had only a single nonfebrile seizure. Many, but not all, of these single seizures were related to nonrecurring infections and the like. A substantial number of the patients would have met the criteria for having epilepsy, except that they were placed on anticonvulsant medications immediately. The prevalence rate has been reported to be even higher in inner-city populations.

Thus far, we have been talking about the risk of having seizures sometime during a person's life. The incidence of seizures (the rate of occurrence of seizures in the population at large during any given year) is much higher in the first year of life and after age 55 years. During the years in between it is approximately 0.5 per 1,000 of population per year (about four new cases each day in a metropolitan population of 2 million, such as Minneapolis/St. Paul). The prevalence of active cases (the percentage of the population who actually have seizures at any given time) is estimated to be between 0.5% and 2%, depending on how the word active is defined. For comparison, the prevalence of insulin-dependent diabetes and classic rheumatoid arthritis is the same, and multiple sclerosis only 0.03%.

DIAGNOSIS

One must make a distinction between a reported experience of a seizure and a diagnosis of a convulsive disorder. It is important to establish that a seizure has actually occurred and to classify that seizure accurately. This information underlies all therapeutic efforts (see the section on Classification, page 7.

Seizure Description

Ordinarily, the physician must depend on a history obtained from the patient and, if possible, the observations of bystanders as to what actually occurred before, during, and after the seizure. Important questions that will help provide clues for classifying the seizure are:

- Did it begin in only one part of the body? (Was it partial?)

- Was there a disturbance of consciousness without complete disruption of motor activity? (Was it complex partial?)
- Did the patient lose awareness without prolonged (more than a few seconds) interruption of normal activity and without engaging in confused, aimless behavior? (Was it an absence attack, ordinarily seen in children?)
- Did the seizure include generalized motor activity with tonic-clonic movements? (Was it a generalized tonic-clonic, formerly called grand mal, seizure?)
- Was this the primary event or was it preceded by a not-so-obvious partial seizure? (Was it a partial seizure secondarily generalized?)
- Was there confusion, sleepiness, or headache after the episode?

Neurological Examination

Anyone who has had an apparent seizure should receive complete physical and neurological examinations and have appropriate laboratory tests. Because seizures may be a symptom of a wide variety of disturbances of the brain, a thorough neurological examination is critical. Seizures may also represent the effect of general metabolic disturbances. Basic laboratory tests, including complete blood cell count, blood glucose measurements, and electrolyte determinations, including calcium, may need to be performed. Consider, also, seizures caused by withdrawal from alcohol and short-acting barbiturates or benzodiazepines. The physician must also be acutely aware of the possibility of underlying disorders such as meningitis, arteriovenous malformation, brain tumor, or hematoma. Special x-ray examinations, including angiography, computerized tomography (CT), and magnetic resonance imaging (MRI) scans are often necessary.

Electroencephalogram Examination

The electroencephalogram (EEG) has a central role in the diagnosis of epilepsy. Interictal seizure activity on the EEG provides strong presumptive evidence that the event was a seizure. However, this is not always the case. The best way to diagnose the presence of seizures and to classify the seizure is to observe, simultaneously, the seizure and the EEG recording. This is not ordinarily possible except in centers especially equipped to carry out long-term video/EEG monitoring. Yet it may be vital if there is confusion about which type of seizure is occurring, about whether the patient has more than one type of seizure, or whether there may be nonepileptic events, psychogenic or physiologic in origin.

An EEG showing no abnormalities does not rule out epilepsy. Paroxysmal abnormalities occur intermittently and may not be easily captured. Repeated EEGs are often needed.

It is often helpful to obtain an EEG during sleep as well as wakefulness. The transition between the alert and sleeping state is often a prime time for epileptiform activity. In fact, some people have epileptiform activity only during sleep, or upon awakening. Because the seizure threshold is lowered in some patients when they are extremely fatigued, sleep deprivation before the sleep EEG is also a useful activating technique.

In a significant number of patients, the EEG will show no abnormality despite repeated recordings. This occurs most commonly in patients with otherwise uncomplicated generalized tonic-clonic seizures, but it can also occur in patients with other types of seizure, especially complex partial seizures. On the other hand, between 1% and 2% of healthy persons without clinically evident seizures have epileptiform discharges on the EEG. Thus the EEG alone neither proves nor rules out epilepsy.

Minimum Conditions for Effective EEG in Seizure Disorders

As a minimum, the following conditions must be met to obtain an adequate EEG for a seizure diagnosis:

- Qualified electroencephalographer (preferably certified by the American Board of Qualification in Electroencephalography, Clinical Neurophysiology, or the Ameri-

can Board of Psychiatry and Neurology with certificate of special competence in clinical neurophysiology)
- Qualified technologist (preferably certified by the American Board of Registration of Electroencephalographic Technologists)
- Adequate recording time
- Patient awake
- Patient asleep
- Sleep deprivation
- Hyperventilation
- Photic stimulation

Know your EEG laboratory. The manner in which the EEG examination is carried out technically and the competence with which it is interpreted cannot be compromised. We depend on the EEG to help make the diagnosis of epilepsy. Failing to diagnose epilepsy promptly leaves the patient at risk for further seizures that may be accompanied by injury or even death. Misdiagnosing epilepsy condemns the patient to taking antiepileptic medications indefinitely and to all the social and psychological handicaps that frequently accompany epilepsy. No one should bear the risk of toxicity and side effects of antiepileptic medicines or be fearful and socially isolated unnecessarily.

Neuropsychological Examination

Specialized neuropsychological testing is often needed in evaluating patients with seizures. These tests not only help to determine the patient's general intelligence and state of brain functioning, but also often help to localize lesions. They rarely need to be performed in simple cases and are usually ordered by a neurologist faced with more complex problems.

Nonepileptic Events (See Chapter 11)

Some people who have never had genuine epileptic seizures may exhibit seizure-like behavior. They are not common in our experience. More often, but still infrequently, patients with genuine seizures will also have nonepileptic events (psychogenic, pseudoseizures, or hysterical seizures). This problem is discussed in detail in Chapter 11.

Psychogenic seizures are not rare. However, not every bizarre seizure is psychogenic. Video EEG monitoring has revealed a greater variety of seizure types than were formerly known. Therefore, the physician must be cautious about making this diagnosis. Because it is often difficult to differentiate between psychogenic and genuine seizures, it may be necessary to refer the patient to a specialized epilepsy center. This referral should be made as early as possible because early intervention is far more effective.

CLASSIFICATION

The distinction between a classification of the epilepsies and a classification of seizures is important. The former classifies epileptic patients by the type of disorder from which they suffer and includes such factors as age, etiology, and prognosis. The latter classifies each individual ictal event.

Classification of the epilepsies has recently been completed by the International League Against Epilepsy (Table 1.1). Two divisions are used. The first separates epilepsies with generalized seizures (so-called generalized epilepsy) from those with partial or focal seizures (so-called localization-related epilepsies). The other division separates those of known etiology (symptomatic or "secondary" epilepsies) from those that are idiopathic (primary) and joined with those that are cryptogenic. By idiopathic we mean no underlying cause other than a possible hereditary predisposition. These idiopathic epilepsies are defined by age-related onset, clinical and EEG characteristics, and a presumed genetic etiology. This is in contrast to the symptomatic epilepsies and syndromes that are the consequence of known or suspected disorders of the central nervous system. The term *cryptogenic* relates to a disorder whose cause

TABLE 1.1 *International Classification of epilepsies and epileptic syndromes*

Localization-related (focal, local, partial) epilepsies and syndromes
    Idiopathic (with age-related onset)
      At present, the following syndromes are established, but more may be identified
        in the future:
      Benign childhood epilepsy with centrotemporal spike
      Childhood epilepsy with occipital paroxysms
      Primary reading epilepsy
    Symptomatic
      Chronic progressive epilepsia partialis continua of childhood
      (Kojewnikow's syndrome)
      Syndromes characterized by seizures with specific modes of precipitation
        (see Chapters 6 and 7 on children, infants)
Generalized epilepsies and syndromes
    Idiopathic (with age-related onset—listed in order of age)
      Benign neonatal familial convulsions
      Benign neonatal convulsions
      Benign myoclonic epilepsy in infancy
      Childhood absence epilepsy (pyknolepsy)
      Juvenile absence epilepsy
      Juvenile myoclonic epilepsy (impulsive petit mal)
      Epilepsy with grand mal (GTCS) seizures on awakening
      Other generalized idiopathic epilepsies not defined above
      Epilepsies with seizures precipitated by specific modes of activation
    Cryptogenic or symptomatic (in order of age)
      West syndrome (infantile spasms, Blitz-Nick-Salaam Krampfe)
      Lennox-Gastaut syndrome
      Epilepsy with myoclonic-astatic seizures
      Epilepsy with myoclonic absences
    Symptomatic
        Nonspecific etiology
          Early myoclonic encephalopathy
          Early infantile epileptic encephalopathy with suppression burst
          Other symptomatic generalized epilepsies not defined above
        Specific syndromes
          Epileptic seizures may complicate many disease states. Under this
            heading are included diseases in which seizures are a presenting or
            predominant feature
Epilepsies and syndromes undetermined whether focal or generalized
    With both generalized and focal seizures
      Neonatal seizures
      Severe myoclonic epilepsy in infancy
      Epilepsy with continuous spike waves during slow wave sleep
      Acquired epileptic aphasia (Landau-Kleffner syndrome)
      Other undetermined epilepsies not defined above
    Without unequivocal generalized or focal features. All cases with generalized
      tonic-clonic seizures in which clinical and EEG findings do not permit classification
      as clearly generalized or localization-related, such as in many cases of
      sleep-grand mal (GTCS) are considered not to have unequivocal generalized or
      focal seizures
Special syndromes
    Situation-related seizures (Gelegenheitsanfalle)
      Febrile convulsions
      Isolated seizures or isolated status epilepticus
      Seizures occurring only when there is an acute metabolic or toxic event due to
        factors such as alcohol, drugs, eclampsia, or nonketotic hyperglycemia

---

is hidden or occult. Cryptogenic epilepsies are often presumed to be symptomatic but there is no etiology identified.

Classification of Seizures

A revised classification of epileptic seizures was adapted in 1981 (Table 1.2). Seizure classification is now based only on clinical observations of seizures and the ictal and interictal EEG expressions. The older classification (1970) included anatomical substrate, etiology, and age factors, but these have been omitted because they are based largely on speculative historical information. Those factors are important, however, in classifying the epilepsies.

Complex partial seizures account for almost two-thirds of the cases of epilepsy. Simple partial seizures and absence seizures are relatively much less common. Uncomplicated tonic-clonic seizures (associated with metabolic derangements, toxins, or withdrawal from toxins and anticonvulsants) are very common. They occur more often as single-seizure episodes as opposed to a recurrent seizure disorder, or epilepsy. Recurrent simple tonic-clonic seizures are a relatively uncommon form of epilepsy.

VIOLENCE AND EPILEPSY

In recent years the association between violence and epilepsy has received a great deal of attention. Books and films have been written around the theme and epilepsy has been used as a defense in murder trials. Articles discussing the relationship between violence and epilepsy are increasing in number in the scientific literature. It is not surprising that some people would ask if an association existed between epilepsy and violence. Violence tends to be an episodic phenomenon, and so are seizures. However, this is reasoning by analogy, which is not good scientific method. A careful review of the literature fails to reveal documented cases of patients acting violently in any directed manner during a seizure. A few patients have been observed on

TABLE 1.2 *International classification of epileptic seizures (1981)*

Partial seizures (beginning focally)
    Simple partial seizures (motor or sensory, including focal motor,
      focal sensory, Jacksonian)
    Complex partial seizures
      With impairment of consciousness at onset
      Simple partial onset, followed by impairment of consciousness
    Partial seizures evolving to generalized tonic-clonic convulsions
      Simple partial evolving to generalized tonic-clonic
      Complex partial evolving to generalized tonic-clonic (including
        those with simple partial onset)
Generalized seizures (convulsive or nonconvulsive)
    First changes indicate initial involvement of both hemispheres;
      consciousness may be impaired, even initially
      Absence seizures
        Impairment of consciousness only
        With automatism, clonic, atonic, or other components
      Atypical absence
    Myoclonic seizures
      Single or multiple myoclonic jerks
      Clonic seizures
    Tonic seizures
    Tonic-clonic seizures
    Atonic seizures
Unclassified (because of incomplete data)

combined video/EEG recording to swear or make a fist during a seizure but no convincing episodes of a directed attack have been reported. On the other hand, many patients with severe, apparently irrational, episodic violence have been studied with no evidence found that the violence was accompanied by activity on the EEG.

From the standpoint of the physician and the patient, there is no reason to believe that violence is associated in any way with ordinary cases of epilepsy. Those patients who have prolonged partial complex seizures in which they wander about may fend off and shove at people who attempt to restrain them. However, if unhindered in their wandering they do not behave violently.

From the standpoint of the lay public, no one need be concerned about being violently attacked by a patient who suffers from epilepsy simply because the patient has seizures. However, some patients with seizures may be violent for other reasons. They should be dealt with in the same manner as a violent person who does not have seizures.

SELECTED READINGS

1. Commission on Classification and Terminology of the International League Against Epilepsy. Proposal for revised classification of epilepsies and epileptic syndromes. *Epilepsia* 1989;30(4):389–399.
2. Commission of Classification and Terminology of the International League Against Epilepsy. Proposal for revised clinical and electroencephalographic classification of epileptic seizures. *Epilepsia* 1981;22:489–501.

2

The Patient With a First Seizure

INITIATING TREATMENT AFTER THE FIRST SEIZURE

When faced with a patient who has had a first seizure, the physician should immediately try to make the proper diagnosis and consider beginning treatment. In general, this is not a wait-and-see situation (except in young children). The second time a seizure occurs, the patient might have an accident and hurt himself or someone else. Furthermore, the social problems accompanying seizures are such that any delay in treatment will only compound the problems that the patient will have to face in society.

Not all seizures are obvious. Seizures frequently involve only part of the brain, and the patient may only shake a hand, twitch the mouth, or have a funny sensation that comes on uncontrollably. The most common form of seizures are complex partial seizures. These patients may experience only a momentary change in consciousness that is hard to distinguish from the absence attacks of childhood. However, they represent a much more serious problem because they indicate that there is focal damage to the brain.

Seizures are often overlooked and delay in diagnosis is common. Only 50% of the patients with epilepsy are diagnosed in the first 6 months of the disorder, and it takes 5 years before 85% are diagnosed by a physician.

SEIZURE THRESHOLD

Every person is capable of having a seizure. For example, hypoxia caused by sudden decompression of an airplane will cause everyone aboard to have a seizure. However, if 10 people are subjected to the same stress, one or two will have seizures much earlier than the others and one or two, much later. Each of us appears to have an inherent seizure threshold, which is largely determined by hereditary factors. This used to be called the seizure diathesis. However, the threshold also fluctuates under the influence of nonspecific factors, for example, going without sleep for prolonged periods, or unusual fatigue. Some people have seizures only as they fall asleep or as they are awakening from deep sleep in the morning.

A low serum calcium level, hormonal changes, such as those of menstruation, inappropriate secretion of antidiuretic hormone, inadequate food intake, water retention, and emotional upset all affect the seizure threshold in most people. In addition, there are often specific brain causes at work, such as an underlying distortion of the brain from a scar, epileptogenic effects of a tumor, or general excitability produced by flashing lights in the 6- to 15-Hz range. Thus, the actual appearance of a seizure is the result of a complex interaction of many factors.

ETIOLOGY

It is important to remember that seizures are a symptom, not a specific disease. Therefore, we must be sure to determine the etiology of the seizure because we may need to treat the primary cause. The etiology is also an important consideration in determining the prognosis.

It is useful to consider some of the causes of seizures. The list that follows is by no means exhaustive, but is designed to stimulate thinking:

- Trauma: seizures may occur acutely at the instant of the trauma, but much more serious are post-traumatic seizures, which may last for years
- Drug withdrawal: barbiturates, benzodiazepines (Valium, Librium, Dalmane), alcohol, anticonvulsants
- Drugs: phenothiazines, antihistamines, amphetamines, low blood sugar produced by insulin and/or tolbutamide, aminophyllin
- Toxins: lead poisoning, arsenic, insecticides, carbon tetrachloride
- Anatomical lesions: brain tumors, arteriovenous malformations, subdural hematomas, old traumatic scars
- Infections: AIDS, syphilis, tuberculosis, fungi, viral encephalitis, bacterial meningitis

EVALUATING THE PATIENT

History and Physical Examination

Whether a physician is a family practitioner or a neurologist, when a new patient comes to your examining room with what is presumed to be a first epileptic seizure it is necessary to carry out a comprehensive evaluation. Critical historical data must be obtained in a precise way, and a general medical and neurological examination performed with competence. It will be necessary to use laboratory examinations judiciously and then carry out an appropriate clinical correlation.

Obtain a careful description of the seizure. The patient may not be aware at all of what happened and the bystanders may provide only snippets of the important information. Nonetheless, talk to the patient's relatives and others who may have witnessed the seizure. Try to document whether or not (a) there was the presence of a subjective warning before the onset of seizure, (b) whether or not there was a disturbance of consciousness, (c) the way in which the clinical behavior associated with the seizure started and what occurred during the course of the seizure, including how long the seizure lasted, and (d) the patient's clinical condition at the end of the clinically obvious seizure. With this information, and by referring to the details in the classification outlined in Chapter 1, it should be possible to develop a preliminary differential diagnosis of whether or not the patient has epilepsy and, if so, what type of seizure has occurred. We are now ready to try to answer two questions: (a) Is the description consistent with that of a seizure and, if so, (b) Does the description tell us whether or not the seizure was partial (focal) or generalized at onset.

Next look for factors that could potentially provoke a seizure in someone who is otherwise not particularly prone to seizures, for example, (a) fever (in children), (b) sleep deprivation, (c) systemic illness or metabolic derangement, (d) abuse or withdrawal from alcohol or other drugs, or (e) flashing lights. Here we are trying to answer the question of whether or not the seizure might have been a reactive one to environmental affects rather than a symptom of an underlying epileptic disorder.

Remember to consider the possibility that what appeared to be a first seizure was in fact the latest in a line of more subtle seizures that had not been recognized. Most patients and their family have no idea what seizures look like and may miss the less obvious ones. It is important to get this information without suggesting to the patient or other observers what the answer should be. It is important to determine whether this is truly a first seizure or whether earlier seizures have occurred, which would tend to point us in the direction of treating early.

Evaluate risk factors. A complete family history should help with questions of a genetic predisposition. Careful past medical history may shed light on whether the patient has acquired some brain damage from trauma, infection, vascular insult, or neoplasm. These would suggest an increased risk for the subsequent development of epilepsy. The interpretation of these risk factors is complex and requires knowledge of current epidemiological studies and many subjective judgments. Serious organic problems will underlie a seizure disorder in a significant number of people, especially after the age of 20 years.

Perform a complete neurological evaluation. Look for focal signs that may indicate an underlying lesion. However, in most cases patients with epilepsy will have a normal neurological examination. Search for other abnormalities in the general medical examination or neurological examination that will suggest underlying systemic or neurological diseases that may require urgent treatment or that may be associated with a higher risk of seizure recurrence.

Imaging and Laboratory Studies

Metabolic studies are ideally performed at the time of the seizure occurrence, when they are most likely to be abnormal. Glucose level, and electrolyte studies, including measurements of calcium and magnesium, are indicated. If the history and examination are suggestive, other metabolic studies such as toxic screens, serologic studies, and vitamin and other nutrient levels may be necessary.

A lumbar puncture (L.P.) is rarely indicated unless the patient presents with signs of acute central nervous system (CNS) inflammations such as fever and stiff neck. Be sure to exclude a potentially dangerous CNS mass lesion. Otherwise the L.P. test has a very low yield. Remember that in children younger than 1 year of age the classic signs of CNS inflammation are often absent.

The electroencephalogram (EEG) examination is indicated nearly always and is by far the most important test. It should be performed in a competent laboratory and should always include sleep and routine activation procedures. The presence of interictal epileptiform abnormalities may indicate an increased risk for seizure recurrence. The EEG often gives evidence regarding the partial or generalized nature of the seizure. Remember that a normal EEG does not exclude epilepsy, nor does an abnormal EEG make the diagnosis of epilepsy. If the first EEG is normal, a second test should be performed after sleep deprivation. Occasionally a third test may provide useful information. After three normal EEGs further interictal EEG studies rarely provide useful information. Preschool children with seizures nearly always have an abnormal EEG. It is important to remember that a child who has an episode, whether awake or asleep, that sounds like it might be a seizure, but who has a normal baseline EEG, is likely to have some other problem.

An examination of the brain structure is almost always indicated. Occasionally it can be postponed in a young child in whom the physician is confident that the diagnosis is that of genetically determined epilepsy. Magnetic resonance imaging (MRI) is the diagnostic tool of choice; computerized tomography (CT) is simply not sensitive enough.

The quality of the MRI examination is critical. The manner in which it is carried out technically and the competence with which it is interpreted cannot be compromised. The lesions that cause epilepsy are often subtle and usually require at least a 1.5T unit, and often special cuts and software manipulations are necessary.

When to Treat a Single Seizure

We never know when the first seizure is a single seizure or the first seizure of chronic epilepsy. Almost 9% of the population will have a seizure sometime in their life; 3%

will have more than one. If we exclude the children with febrile seizures, half the people who have one seizure will have another sometime in their life.

Do treat:

- A patient with a clear-cut epileptic focus on the EEG
- A patient with an MRI or CT lesion
- A patient with an abnormal neurological examination suggesting brain damage
- A patient with a history of epilepsy in parents and especially siblings (except simple febrile seizures)
- A patient with a history of previous brain infection, or head injury with loss of consciousness
- A patient with active infection in the brain (encephalitis, meningitis, abscess)
- A patient with status epilepticus as the first seizure

Possibly treat:

- Uncomplicated "single seizure" if history suggests the possibility that one occurred earlier
- A single seizure in someone at risk if a second seizure occurs (driving, employment, living alone, etc.)

Don't treat:

- A single seizure from alcohol withdrawal
- A single seizure from drug abuse
- Simple febrile seizures
- Epilepsy with centrotemporal spikes
- Seizures from sleep deprivation
- Seizures with acute illness that is responding to treatment (fever, hypoglycemia, dehydration, water logging)
- A single uncomplicated seizure in a child under age 6 years
- A single seizure that does not sound like epilepsy in a patient with psychological or social issues suggesting fertile grounds for psychogenic seizures

Listening to Questions from the Patient

When someone has a first seizure, the physician should be prepared to listen to the questions: Why me? Why did it happen? Will I die? What could I have done to prevent it? When asked by a parent or spouse, these questions often reflect the guilt that is natural under the circumstances. Parents often believe that they should have been aware of all dangers and should have protected their child. Frequently, of course, there are no answers to the questions.

Providing Information

The physician should be prepared to provide a good deal of general information about epilepsy and as much as possible about the specific case. How did it happen? Why did it happen to our child or my husband? Why can't you cure it? These are all natural questions. Coping with the problems of epilepsy goes beyond these questions, however. The additional aspects must be addressed directly by the physician. Speak directly to the patient. It may be necessary to talk separately to the spouse and other family members even if they were in the room at the same time. If the patient is a child, even if that child is only 3 or 4 years old, speak directly to the child. Give the patient of any age a chance to express their fears, concerns, and desire for information.

The patient and all concerned will need to know the name and the type of seizure, what the seizure looks like, what kind of behavior is likely before, during, and after a seizure, what first aid should be given (see Appendix), and what kind of behavior is inappropriate. The distinction between a single seizure and the diagnosis of epilepsy, implying the presence of recurrent seizures, is important. Single seizures occur twice as commonly as epilepsy in the general population. Ideally we would like not to treat the patient with single seizures and to treat the patient who is likely to have a recurrence. The scientific literature pro-

TABLE 2.1. *Recurrent risk from a single seizure at 1, 3, and 5 years*

Description	1 Year (%)	3 Years (%)	5 Years (%)
No previous history	10	24	29
History of CNS insult	26	41	48
Sibling with seizures	29		46
No sibling history	9		26
EEG pattern of generalized spikes and waves	15		58
Normal/nonspecific EEG	9		26
Previous acute seizure with illness	10		39
Previous acute seizure without illness	60		80
Todd's postictal paresis	41		75
Status epilepticus or multiple seizures at onset	37		56

Data supplied by W. A. Hauser.
CNS, central nervous system; EEG, electroencephalogram.

vides some guidelines for estimating the risk (Table 2.1). However, in the best case scenario, the risk occurrence will still be about 25% to 35%. The patient and family members will also want to know when a seizure is a medical emergency and when they should simply call for reassurance, whom the patient should call and how, and how to avoid unnecessary trips to the emergency room. The physician should be sure that the patient knows why medications are used, the generic and trade names of the drugs prescribed, the dosage prescribed, the medication side effects, and what to do in case of a missed dose. Last, but equally important to the patient's well being, is making sure that she knows how to cope with the knowledge of having seizures and to put things in a proper perspective. Be sure to discuss the issue of driving and work restrictions to limit the risk of injury in the event of recurrent seizures.

PATIENT'S SELF-MANAGEMENT

If the seizures are not immediately controlled, it is usually necessary for the patient to keep a careful diary of what type of seizures occur, when they occur, and when she takes her medication. In this way, the physician can reconstruct what has happened during the intervals between office visits. The patient also comes to understand how her behavior has a good deal to do with the success of treatment. There have been a variety of methods developed for keeping diaries, some quite elaborate, others consisting of nothing more than a simple notebook. The patient's diary shown in the Appendix has been found to be quite useful and the tear-out sheet may be reproduced and adopted for use.

The therapeutic aim is a complete halt to the seizures. One to two seizures a year is too many. We wish to avoid the disability that accompanies even the occasional seizure. Often, the patient will develop a poor self-image, the community will be intolerant, and employment and recreation will become difficult.

Everyone who has a first seizure is extremely anxious. Even if the patient denies any concern, her anxiety needs to be addressed directly. The best way to deal with anxiety is to provide a lot of facts, both about epilepsy in general and about the patient's own personal situation. Try to maximize the areas that the patient can control to minimize dependency and provide emotional support.

Everyone who has a seizure is afraid, if they have any self-awareness at all. Relatively few express the fear openly. It is helpful for the physician to address the fear directly and provide the patient with an opportunity to express it. This is particularly true regarding the fear of dying in a seizure. This fear is almost universal and quite rational.

It is important to evaluate the patient's coping, defense, and reward mechanisms. Many patients approach problems in a passive and inadequate fashion, coping no better with seizures than they do with other stresses of daily living.

When just told of the diagnosis of epilepsy the average patient closes her ears and doesn't hear another word. A second visit should be scheduled soon to repeat the essential medical information. A third visit will be needed to begin to address the key psychosocial issues that face the patient. The physician or appropriate staff member (nurse, social worker) should begin the task of helping the patient set realistic goals for the future. For example, what will be the effect of not being able to drive for at least 6 months, perhaps permanently? Certain occupations (airplane pilot, bus or truck driver) will not be possible. The choice of job may be influenced by the availability of appropriate health insurance. Most patients undergo at least a moderate situational depression. The patient may benefit from reading a copy of my book *Living Well With Epilepsy* (Demos, NY 1990).

ADVISING FAMILIES ABOUT FIRST AID

A first seizure can be a frightening experience for the patient and for those nearby. Family members will need to know what to do if another seizure occurs. Complete first-aid instructions are given in Chapter 9 and the Appendix and may be copied from the book. Handy wallet-sized cards are available free of charge (in small quantities) from MINCEP® Epilepsy Care, 5775 Wayzata Blvd., Minneapolis, MN 55416.

Antiepileptic Medication Treatment

3

GENERAL PRINCIPLES OF TREATMENT

Epilepsy can rarely be cured but it can usually be controlled. When seizures are produced by a brain tumor, hematoma, or arteriovenous malformation, the basic treatment is twofold: first, the use of antiepileptic medicines to stop the seizures and, second, surgical removal of the lesion, if indicated. Often, an operation will stop the seizures as well.

Antiepileptic medicines are used first in nearly all cases. When they do not bring about complete control of the seizures, or do so only with unacceptable toxicity, then surgical treatment should be considered (see Chapter 13).

Control of seizures is paramount in the treatment of epilepsy, but it is only part of the treatment. The behavioral, social, and economic consequences of having uncontrolled seizures are enormous. Substantial amounts of emotional support and the involvement of a team of nurses, social workers, vocational counselors, and other health professionals is often necessary. Even patients with relatively simple problems, whose seizures are immediately controlled with small doses of anticonvulsants, often have serious questions or doubts. These will cause long-standing anxiety if not dealt with early and appropriately.

Proper Medication

Antiepileptic medicines are effective in preventing seizures only as long as they are taken as prescribed. If the patient takes the medications irregularly, or not at all, seizure activity may begin again. If a significant loss or gain of body weight has occurred or if the patient juggles dosage on his own, a deterioration of seizure control or scholastic or athletic performance may occur.

Starting Anticonvulsant Medication

The general principles are to try one drug, beginning with one-third or one-half the recommended dose, gradually increase the dosage to the point of toxicity, and change drugs if toxicity develops without seizure control or if *serious* side effects occur. Starting with a small dose and gradually increasing the dose minimizes toxicity, thus avoiding an unpleasant and frightening experience that may lead the patient to refuse to take an effective medicine. Idiosyncratic side effects are of particular concern. The physician may find it useful to keep a diary for each patient, such as the one shown in the Appendix, in which medications and plasma drug levels are correlated with seizure frequency. The form may be reproduced and adopted for the reader's use.

Therapy with antiepileptic medicines should be based on the rational choice of a single drug known to be effective for the particular seizure type and to produce the fewest side effects. The choice of a single agent among the drugs active for the specific seizure type depends on several factors, including:

- Previous history of drug allergies

- Tolerance of side effects
- Childbearing potential
- Age of patient
- Economic circumstances

Initiate the drug at the recommended daily dosage and evaluate serum drug levels after 5 to 8 half-lives (or 3–4 weeks if the patient is not having seizures). If seizures recur and compliance has been verified, increase the dosage until the patient either achieves seizure control or begins to experience mild toxicity. At that point, consider the addition of a second antiepileptic medicine. Most patients with seizures should be able to achieve control with a single drug.

Linking Seizure Type to Choice of Drug

The most commonly used antiepileptic medicines (AEMs) and the seizure types for which they are effective are shown in Table 3.1. Three new AEMs have been recently approved by the FDA: felbamate, gabapentin, and lamotrigine. They are listed in the table. All three offer advantages over some of the well-established AEMs, especially in terms of side effects.

Establishing Therapeutic Range of Serum Drug Level

A serious misconception is the belief that *blood levels of antiepileptic medicines* should lie within specified "therapeutic" or "normal" ranges. These values, however, represent only the ranges of serum drug levels in which most patients experience control of seizures with few side effects. There are many patients who need higher levels for seizure control and who do not experience serious side effects. Conversely, others may experience unpleasant side effects at levels within the "therapeutic" range. Clinical experience

TABLE 3.1. *Preferred antiepileptic drug by seizure type*

Seizure type	First line	Second line	Contraindicated
Generalized absence	Zarontin Depakote		Phenobarbital Mebarol Mysoline
Generalized tonic-clonic	Dilantin Tegretol Depakote	Phenobarbital Mysoline Felbatol Lamictal Neurontin	
Tonic drop attack	Felbatol Depakote Klonopin	Phenobarbital Mysoline	Phenobarbital Mebarol Mysoline
Partial simple	Dilantin Tegretol Lamictal Phenobarbital	Mysoline Klonopin Neurontin Felbatol	
Complex partial	Dilantin Tegretol Lamictal Neurontin	Phenobarbital Mysoline Depakote Klonopin Felbatol	
Secondarily generalized tonic-clonic	Dilantin Tegretol Lamictal Neurontin Depakote	Phenobarbital Mysoline Klonopin Felbatol	

Felbatol is a potent effective AED. It is listed as a second line drug only because it has been reported (08/01/94) by the FDA to have a 20-50 times higher incidence of aplastic anemia than the baseline rate in the general population.

and judgment must be used in conjunction with monitoring of serum antiepileptic medicine levels. Dosages must be individualized.

Dosage Interval

The dosage interval for a given drug should be chosen with its half-life in mind. A good rule of thumb is that the dosage interval should not exceed the half-life. Thus, in theory, Dilantin can be given once a day, generic phenytoin must be given three times a day, and Depakene must be given at least three and often four or five times a day, whereas Depakote may be given twice a day.

Missed Doses

Everyone occasionally forgets to take a dose of medicine. Many patients worry unduly about this. For nearly all but the most rapidly eliminated anticonvulsants, an occasional missed dose can be made up by taking it within the same 24-hour period. For this reason, many patients find it convenient to put their medication into an egg carton or plastic pill box with divided compartments. A number of commercially made dosage boxes are available. Patients can set out a week's supply of pills and glance at the appropriate day's box each night before going to bed. Any pills that are left over can be taken at that time. Rarely will these patients experience difficulty with side effects from an *occasional* doubled dose. Those who do will have to work out an interval schedule that avoids difficulty.

Stopping Antiepileptic Medication in Adults

Although some people eventually become seizure-free after many years, patients should be prepared to take medication for a long time. There are specific situations in which the patient and the physician may wisely consider stopping anticonvulsants:

1. Concern about taking medicine: If a patient has been seizure-free for at least 2 years (preferably 5–10 years) and is particularly anxious about taking drugs, it is reasonable to consider a trial withdrawal. However, inform the patient that about one-fourth to one-half the patients will have a recurrence of seizures within a year, especially if they have neurological findings, an abnormal MRI, or continuing epileptiform activity on the EEG.

2. Ineffective drug levels: It is reasonable to stop anticonvulsant medications if the patient has been seizure-free and blood levels of the drugs are so low as to indicate that the patient has not been compliant.
3. Pregnancy (see section on pregnancy about prophylaxis for teratogenicity): If the patient experiences only rare seizures and she is concerned about possible birth defects, it is reasonable to consider a trial period without anticonvulsant medication before she becomes pregnant. The risk of teratogenicity is in the first trimester. *Do not stop medication after pregnancy has been diagnosed.* It is too late to protect the fetus, and the mother will suffer a needless risk.
4. Long seizure-free period: If the patient has been seizure-free for a long time (10 years or more) and is willing to risk losing a driver's license if seizures recur, it is reasonable to stop anticonvulsant medication.

See Chapter 6 for special information about stopping AEMs in children.

Uncontrolled or Intractable Seizures

If the patient is not seizure-free and is experiencing medication toxicity, consider a referral to a specialized epilepsy center (see Chapter 12). All these patients will benefit from the combination of skills available there and some of them will become surgical candidates. The longer patients have uncontrolled seizures, the harder it is to treat them successfully.

USE OF ANTIEPILEPTIC MEDICINES

A Method for the Use of Antiepileptic Medicines

1. Initiate therapy with one medicine. Choose one that is most likely to be effective for the seizure type (see Table 3.1) and is most suitable for the patient.
2. Start with a low dose to avoid sudden unpleasant side effects that will frighten the patient away from a useful agent.

3. Use an adequate dosage of the chosen medicine. Increase the dosage to attain and maintain therapeutic serum levels. Allow adequate time for the medicine to achieve a steady-state level, and verify that the level is within the usual effective range. Each medicine requires four to five times its serum half-life to reach a steady state. Be familiar with the individual pharmacokinetics of the medicine you prescribe.

4. Advise the patient to keep a seizure diary (see Appendix) to assist in evaluating the effectiveness of the regimen. Increase the dose to the point of toxicity if seizures persist.

5. Evaluate compliance, especially if the medicine does not appear to be effective. Monitor plasma drug levels and review with the patient the method for remembering to take medication.

6. If the first medicine is not effective at toxic levels, add a second medicine. Decrease the first medicine gradually after the second medicine has produced control.

7. If the first medicine is only partially effective, increase the dose. If toxic symptoms occur, reduce the dose to the next highest one at which the patient did not have unacceptable side effects. Now add a second medicine and gradually increase the dose to attain control. Continue the first medicine for awhile. Because of drug interactions it will be necessary to check the serum level of the first medicine also. The second medicine also should be pushed to the point of toxicity if necessary. If the patient becomes seizure-free, withdraw the first medicine gradually in order to treat with only one medicine if possible.

8. Schedule doses for maximum anticonvulsant effect and minimum side effects (Table 3.2): (a) give medicine at intervals no longer than one half-life; (b) give medicine with sedative effects at bedtime; and (c) give medicine to achieve peak levels at the specific time of day when the patient consistently has seizures.

Guidelines for the Patient and Family

When initiating therapy, and periodically during a long-term treatment, discuss the medicine in detail with the patient and his family. Emphasize the following points:

- General safety of medicines when taken as prescribed
- Name and dose of each tablet, capsule, or liquid prescribed
- Side effects requiring evaluation by the physician
- Methods for remembering to take the medicine regularly

TABLE 3.2. *Side effects of the most commonly used antiepileptic medicines*

Drug	U.S. trade name	Common side effects with monotherapy
Carbamazepine	Tegretol	Sedation, diplopia, diarrhea
Clonazepam	Klonopin	Sedation, dizziness
Ethosuximide	Zarontin	Drowsiness, hyperactivity, nausea
Felbamate	Felbatol	Insomnia, headache, weight loss, nausea, dizziness
Gabapentin	Neurontin	Somnolence, fatigue, dizziness, ataxia
Lamotrigine	Lamictal	Diplopia, drowsiness, headache, nausea
Mephobarbital	Mebaral	Drowsiness, lethargy, dizziness
Phenobarbital		Drowsiness, lethargy, dizziness, hyperactivity
Phenytoin	Dilantin	Disturbance of equilibrium, hirsutism, gingival hyperplasia, acne, anemia, double vision
Primidone	Mysoline	Drowsiness, appetite loss, irritability, nausea, vomiting, dizziness, loss of coordination, tremor
Valproic acid	Depakene Depakote	Indigestion, nausea, increased appetite, sedation, dizziness, hair loss, tremor

On August 1, 1994, the FDA reported that patients taking Felbatol had an incidence of aplastic anemia 20-50 times higher than the baseline rate in the general public.

- Problems with missed doses and possible corrective steps
- Necessity for regular blood tests
- Procedure for obtaining prescription refills to avoid running out of medication
- Risk of status epilepticus if medication is abruptly discontinued

Side Effects

Side effects related to high plasma levels can be ameliorated by dividing the total daily dosage into more frequent smaller doses and by taking the dose with meals or at bedtime.

Side effects related to hypersensitivity include:

- Rash
- Blood dyscrasia/Aplastic anemia
- Gastrointestinal symptoms, especially diarrhea
- Drug-induced systemic lupus erythematosus
- Immunological disorders
- Lymphadenopathy
- Hepatitis
- Stevens-Johnson syndrome
- Nephrotic syndrome (trimethadione)

Long-term side effects include:

- Anemia (folic acid deficiency)
- Gingival hypertrophy (phenytoin)
- Skeletal abnormalities (rickets, phenytoin)
- Endocrinological disorders

Side effects during pregnancy are:

- Teratogenicity
- Coagulation defects in the neonate

Recommended Guidelines for Laboratory Studies

1. Perform baseline studies before beginning anticonvulsant therapy, including complete blood cell count, platelets and differential, and liver function tests
2. Repeat these every 3 months for 1 year, and then once a year thereafter (every 6 months with carbamazepine)
3. The laboratory tests should be repeated each time an additional antiepileptic medicine is prescribed
4. If it becomes necessary to discontinue a drug abruptly because of a reaction, hospitalize the patient and start an alternative drug to avoid an increase in seizure frequency. The new drug may need to be introduced quickly; consider a loading dose and take precautions against side effects. A flurry of withdrawal seizures can usually be controlled with Lorazepam

Quality Control Laboratory Program

Concentrations of drugs in blood should be measured accurately. To ensure the accuracy of these determinations, there is a national quality control program for laboratory testing. Ask your laboratory whether it is enrolled in the Therapeutic Drug Monitoring Program of the American Association for Clinical Chemistry and, if so, how well it scores.

Measuring Antiepileptic Medicine Concentrations

Antiepileptic medicine concentrations should be measured:

- To monitor the patient's adherence to the dosage schedule
- To check for changes in the patient's metabolism affecting drug half-life and serum drug level
- Before modifying dosage
- After initiating or modifying antiepileptic medicine therapy (measure after steady state has been achieved)

- When signs and symptoms of drug intoxication occur
- If seizures recur in a previously well-controlled patient
- If medical problems develop, especially those involving hepatic, renal, or hematopoietic function
- If the patient takes other medication that affects the elimination of antiepileptic medicines
- Once a year in well-controlled patients

Compliance

Patients fail to take medications regularly for a wide variety of reasons. These are discussed in Chapter 10. A reliable way to check for compliance is to measure antiepileptic medicine levels two or three times at the same time of day (assuming the patient takes medications at regular times each day), especially when the patient isn't expecting it. Variations of more than plus or minus 20% indicate noncompliance.

ANTIEPILEPTIC MEDICINES COMMONLY USED FOR ADULTS

The proper dosage for each patient will depend on many factors, including age, weight, severity of the epileptogenic process, associated CNS disease, and hepatic or renal function. The drugs are listed alphabetically by generic name. Any drug can cause idiosyncratic or hypersensitivity reactions in skin, blood, or bowel.

Carbamazepine (Tegretol and Others)

Indications: Simple partial seizures, complex partial seizures, generalized tonic-clonic seizures
Average daily dose:
    Initial: 200 mg b.i.d., increase gradually
    Maintenance: 15 mg/kg, divided into three or more doses

Formulation: 200 mg tablets, 100 mg chewable tablets, suspension 100 mg/5 ml
Metabolism: Hepatic conversion to epoxide and other metabolites
Serum half-life: 24 hr initially, then 12 ± 6 hr after auto induction
Time to achieve steady state: 2 to 4 days
Effective blood level: usually >4 µg/ml
Toxic level (dose-related side effects): usually begins to appear above 8 µg/ml
Note: Common pharmacokinetic interactions include:
1. Autoinduction reduces half-life to 12 hr after 2 weeks of monotherapy
2. Carbamazepine level drops, epoxide metabolite level increases with simultaneous use of felbatol, lamotrigine, phenytoin, and valproic acid
3. If patient on polytherapy and toxic, measure the 10,11-epoxide levels as well
4. Different manufacturers supply tablets that vary in bioavailability; stick to one brand

Common side effects: Drowsiness, dizziness, blurred vision, difficulty in thinking, diarrhea

Clonazepam (Klonopin)

Indications: Myoclonic seizures, useful as a secondary drug for complex partial seizures and tonic seizures
Average daily dose:
  Initial: 0.5 mg b.i.d., increase as tolerated over the next several weeks
  Maintenance: 1 to 20 mg, divided into two to four doses
Formulation: 0.5 mg, 1 mg, and 2 mg tablets
Metabolism: Hepatic
Serum half-life: 27 ± 5 hr
Time to achieve steady state: 4 to 5 days
Effective blood level: Blood level measurements rarely helpful

Note: Increase dosage slowly to avoid excessive sedation
Common side effects: Drowsiness, difficulty in thinking

Ethosuximide (Zarontin)

Indications: Absence seizures only
Average daily dose: 750 to 2,000 mg, may be divided into two doses
Formulation: 250 mg capsules, syrup 250 mg/5 ml
Metabolism: Hepatic
Serum half-life: 30 ± 12 hr
Time to achieve steady state: 5 to 10 days
Effective blood level: >40 μg/ml
Toxic level (dose-related side effects): >150 μg/ml
Common side effects: Drowsiness

Felbamate (Felbatol)

Indications: Complex partial seizures, drop attacks, tonic-clonic, and atypical absence seizures in Lennox-Gasteux syndrome
Contraindications: None
Average daily dose: 1,200 to 3,600 mg per day or more if necessary
Formulation: Tablets of 400 and 600 mg, suspension 600 mg/5 ml
Metabolism: Hydroxilation and conjugation in the liver
Serum half-life: 14 hr
Time to achieve steady state: 3 days
Effective blood level: Not known, tentatively greater than 50 μg/ml
Toxic level (dose-related side effects): Not known
Common side effects: Insomnia, weight loss, headache, decreased appetite, dizziness, fatigue. A rash may be seen if the patient is also taking Depakote

Felbatol is associated with two major allergic complications. Patients taking Felbatol have a 1/2000 chance per year (estimated) of developing aplastic anemia (with a 25% death rate) and a 1/5000 chance per year (estimated) of developing liver failure (with a 50% death rate). Physicians should prescribe Felbatol only for patients who have a serious seizure problem and who have not responded to safer AED's.

Gabapentin (Neurontin)

Indications: Gabapentin has been approved as an add-on supplementary agent for patients with partial and/or secondary generalized tonic-clonic seizures
Contraindications: None
Average daily dose: 1,800 to 3,600 mg per day or more. No more than 600 mg in any one dose
Formulation: Capsules of 100, 300, and 400 mg
Metabolism: Renal secretion as the parent compound
Serum half-life: 5 to 7 hr
Time to achieve steady state: 36 hr
Effective blood level: Not known
Toxic level (dose-related side effects): Not known (very low toxicity under any circumstances)
Common side effects: Somnolence, fatigue, dizziness, ataxia

Lamotrigene (Lamictal)

At the time that this book was written, a new drug application had been filed for lamotrigene, but it has not yet been approved by the FDA in the United States and a package insert is not available. This information is based on the experience with lamotrigine at MINCEP® Epilepsy Care since 1988.

Indications: Partial complex and/or secondary generalized tonic-clonic seizures
Contraindications: None

Average daily dose: 300 to 600 mg or more per day, children about 50% of this

Formulation: 25 mg, 50 mg, 100 mg, 150 mg, and 250 mg

Metabolism: Predominantly in the liver and secreted as a glucuronide

Serum half-life: 14 hr (if patient is taking Depakote, 60 hr)

Time to achieve steady state: 2 days

Effective blood level: 1 to 3 μg/ml

Toxic level (dose-related side effects): Not known

Common side effects: Drowsiness, dizziness, headache, and nausea. A rash is commonly seen if the patient is also taking Depakote

Phenobarbital

Indications: Partial seizures, generalized tonic-clonic seizures

Contraindications: Absence seizures, atypical absence seizures, and drop attacks

Average daily dose: 90 to 240 mg (1–3 mg/kg), may be given in one or divided doses

Formulation: 15 mg, 30 mg, 60 mg, and 100 mg tablets, elixir 400 mg/100 ml

Metabolism: Hydroxylated by the liver, but a significant amount is excreted unchanged by the kidneys

Serum half-life: 96 ± 12 hr

Time to achieve steady state: 14 to 21 days

Effective blood level: >20 μg/ml

Toxic level (dose-related side effects): >40 μg/ml

Common side effects: Drowsiness, difficulty thinking, loss of balance, hyperactivity

Phenytoin (Dilantin*)

Indications: Partial seizures, complex partial seizures, generalized tonic-clonic seizures

Average daily dose: 200 to 400 mg (4–6 mg/kg), divided into two or more doses

Formulation: 30 mg and 100 mg capsules; 50 mg chewable tablets, scored (bioavailability different from capsules); 30 mg/5 ml and 125 mg/5 ml suspension (unreliable, not recommended for routine use)

Metabolism: Hydroxylated by liver (dose-level relationship is not linear; small increases in dose may result in large increases in plasma level)

Serum half-life: 24 ± 12 hr

Time to achieve steady state: 5 to 10 days

Effective blood level: >10 µg/ml

Toxic level (dose-related side effects): >20 µg/ml

Note: Because absorption and half-life vary among formulations of different manufacturers, consistently use one brand. Previous generic name: diphenylhydantoin

Common side effects: Hirsutism, acne, dizziness, difficulty thinking

---

*A delayed absorption form, not equivalent to rapidly absorbed generic phenytoin.

Primidone (Mysoline)

Indications: Partial motor seizures, complex partial seizures, generalized tonic-clonic seizures

Contraindications: Absence seizures, atypical absence seizures, and drop attacks

Average daily dose:
  Initial: 125 mg b.i.d., increase very gradually
  Maintenance: 750 to 1,500 mg, divided into three or more doses

Formulation: 50 mg and 250 mg tablets, scored. Suspension 250 mg/5 ml.

Metabolism: Hepatic conversion to phenobarbital and phenylethylmalonamide (PEMA)

Serum half-life: 12 ± 6 hr (96 ± 12 hr for phenobarbital)

Time to achieve steady state: 4 to 7 days (14–21 days for phenobarbital)

Effective blood level: >5 µg/ml

Toxic level (dose-related side effects): <12 µg/ml; dizziness and nausea may occur unless initial dosage is low (50 mg t.i.d.) and gradually increased

Note: Because primidone is primarily metabolized to phenobarbital, also check plasma phenobarbital level. Unexplained toxicity may be related to elevated PEMA level

Common side effects: Drowsiness, difficulty thinking, nausea, psychotic reactions

Valproic Acid (Depakene/Depakote)

Indications: Absence seizures, generalized tonic-clonic seizures, may be helpful in complex partial seizures

Average daily dose: 750 to 2,000 mg (15–30 mg/kg), divided into three or more doses

Formulation: Depakene 250 mg capsules, 250 mg/5 ml syrup. Depakote: 125, 250, 500 mg tablets, 125 mg "sprinkle capsules"

Metabolism: Hepatic

Serum half-life: 12 ± 6 hr

Time to achieve steady state: 2 to 4 days

Effective blood level: 20 to 40 µg/ml (trough); 50–90 µg/ml (peak, 1 hr after dose)

Toxic level (dose-related side effects): >90 µg/ml

Common side effects: Nausea, weight gain, hair loss, diarrhea, difficulty thinking, drowsiness

POLYPHARMACY AND DRUG INTERACTIONS

All antiepileptic medications affect and/or are affected by other medications taken at the same time, except, perhaps, Neurontin. This is even truer when two antiepileptic drugs are taken together. Among the advantages of monotherapy is that taking only one medicine minimizes these interactions, reduces toxicity, and simplifies dosing.

Table 3.3 outlines the major and most common interactions of antiepileptic drugs with other drugs. Table 3.4 addresses the interactions between antiepileptic drugs. Table 3.5 lists investigational drugs coming to market.

Although many of these interactions are predictable, there will be an increased need to measure antiepileptic drug concentrations and the concentration of certain metabolites when the patient takes more than one medicine.

EXAMPLES OF ANTIEPILEPTIC MEDICINE TREATMENT

Woman Taking Contraceptives

A 23-year-old woman has partial complex with secondary generalized tonic-clonic seizures. Her weight is 132 lb (60 kg). She is also taking oral contraceptives. Potential drug choices are phenytoin, carbamazepine, phenobarbital, primidone, felbamate, gabapentin, and lamotrogine.

1. *Phenytoin:*   You choose phenytoin because it is inexpensive and relatively nonsedating. The first target dose prescribed was 5 mg/kg, which is a daily dosage of 300 mg. One month later, the serum phenytoin level is 4 μg/ml, much lower than expected. She may be exhibiting rapid metabolism, noncompliance, or poor absorption. Because poor compliance is a frequent problem, you stress the need to take the drug as prescribed. You check serum drug blood levels 1 week later and again 2 weeks later. If all three levels are within plus or minus 20%, the patient is most likely compliant. If so, the dosage should be increased. This patient may be rapidly metabolizing phenytoin because of the effects of alcohol, oral contraceptives, or other drugs. Note also that antiepileptic medicines may decrease the effectiveness of oral contraceptives by increasing their metabolism.

   The hepatic enzymes that metabolize phenytoin are saturated at plasma concentrations of 10 to 15 μg/ml. A

TABLE 3.3 *Antiepileptic medicines: interaction with other (nonepileptic) drugs.*

AEM	Drug Added	Blood level (concentration) of AEM	Blood level (concentration) of other drug
Carbamazepine	Propoxyphene	↑	
	Cimetidine	↑	
	Isoniazid	↑	
	Erythromycin	↑	
	Warfarin	↔	↓
	Theophylline	↔	↓
	Doxycycline	↔	↓
Phenobarbital	Oral contraceptives	↔	↓ efficacy
Primidone	Quinidine	↔	↓
	Tricyclicse	↔	↓
	Corticosteriods	↔	↓
	Chlorpromazine	↔	↓
	Furosemide	↔	↓ renal response
Phenytoin	Antacids	↓	
	Disulfiram	↑	
	Isoniazid	↑	
	Chlorasmphenicol	↑	
	Propoxyphene	↑	
	Cimetidine	↑	
	Ethanol	↓	
	Oral contraceptives	↔	↓ efficacy
	Bishydroxycoumarin	↔	↓ anticoagulation effect
	Quinidine	↔	↓
	Vitamin D	↔	↓
	Folic Acid	↔	↓
Valproic acid	Salicylates	↑ free concentration	

NB Modified from DiPiro JT. *Psychopharmacology*. Elsevier: Amsterdam, 1989.

small increase in dosage at these levels will result in a large increase in serum drug level. Thus, if she had a level of 13 µg/ml with a daily dosage of 400 mg the next increase should be 30 mg, which would most probably give a level of 18 to 20 µg/ml.

TABLE 3.4 *Antiepileptic medicines: interactions with other antiepileptic medicines.*

AEM	Additional AEM	Effect	N.B.
Carbamazepine	Phenobarbital	↓	
	Phenytoin	↓	10,11-epoxide
	Primidone	↓	
	Felbamate	↓	↑ epoxide
Phenobarbital	Phenytoin	↑, ↓, or ↔	
	Valproic acid	↑	30-50% increase
Phenytoin	Carbamazepine	↓	
	Methsuccimide	↑	occasionally
	Valproic acid	↓ total	↑ unbound (↑ toxicity)
	Felbamate	↑	↓ PHT dose 20%
	Vigabatrine	↓	Investigational drug; ↑ PHT dose 20-40%
Primidone	Phenytoin	↑	PR may go ↑, ↓ or ↔
	Carbamazepine	↔	PEMA may ↑ PB may ↑
Valproic Acid	Carbamazepine	↓	
	Phenobarbital	↓	
	Primidone	↓	
	Phenytoin	↓ total	↑ unbound
	Felbamate	↑ total	↑ 2 'ene metabolite
Lamotrigine	Valproic Acid	↑ half life and level	Reduce lamotrigine dose by 50-70%

2. *Carbamazepine:*   You choose carbamazepine because it does not produce gingival hypertrophy. However, it costs more and has a higher risk for hematological and neural tube complications (which can largely be avoided by prescribing 1–4 mg folic acid daily). The final dosage may need to be higher than the initial dosage because carbamazepine induces its own metabolism. Its short half-life is associated with large daily fluctuations in concentration, so time of blood sampling relative to the dosage must be constant for proper interpretation of serum drug levels.

Table 3.5 *Investigational antiepileptic medicines**

Drug Name	Pharmaceutical Company	Mechanism of Action	Notes
Flunarizine	Ciba Geigy	Unknown	Marketed in Europe
Lamotrigine	Burroughs Wellcome	Unknown	NDA filed; Marketed in England, Canada
Oxcarbazepine	Ciba Geigy	Unknown	Marketed in Europe
Remacemide	Fisons	?Block excitatory amino acids	
Tiagabine	Abbott	Block gaba uptake	
Vigabatrin	Marion Merrill Dow	Gabatransminase blocker	Marketed in Europe
Zonisamide	Dainippon	Unknown	Marketed in Japan

*At the time this chapter was prepared (summer 1994), there were an unusually large number of new antiepileptic medicines undergoing clinical investigation. The above look promising. An NDA for lamotrigine has already been submitted to the FDA.

3. *Phenobarbital:* You choose phenobarbital because it is very inexpensive and has the least amount of idiosyncratic reactions, even though it may cause lethargy and depression. Its long half-life is useful if the patient has problems with compliance. The initial daily dosage is 3 mg/kg, and you warn the patient about phenobarbital's interaction with alcohol and sedatives.

Man Receiving Combination Drug Therapy

A 43-year-old man, 220 lb (100 kg), with generalized tonic-clonic seizures, is receiving phenytoin (300 mg/day) and phenobarbital (90 mg/day) but he is still having one seizure every 9 months. His serum drug levels are 2 μg/ml for phenytoin and 6 µg/ml for phenobarbital. He is known to be compliant.

1. *Phenytoin:*   The phenytoin dosage is much too low for his body weight and the concentration is not likely to be effective. You should increase the dosage to 6 mg/kg and aim for serum phenytoin levels of 10 to 15 µg/ml.
2. *Phenobarbital:*   Phenobarbital level is far too low. Discontinue and try for control on phenytoin monotherapy.

DENTAL PROBLEMS WITH ANTIEPILEPTIC MEDICINES

The only antiepileptic medicine that causes substantial mouth and gum problems is phenytoin. Phenytoin is one of the oldest, least expensive, and most effective drugs for controlling seizures; therefore, it is in very wide use. Common side effects are swelling, overgrowth, and irritation of the gums. Whether this becomes a serious problem will depend on the dental care habits of the patient.

Good dental care habits can prevent the gum problems associated with phenytoin. Once the complications occur, they are much more difficult and expensive to treat. A patient taking phenytoin should begin a comprehensive dental care program with a visit to the dentist for an evaluation and correction of present problems. The dentist should clean the teeth and fill any cavities present. The dentist may recommend an acrylic resin sealant to fill in pits and fissures in hard-to-get-at places where it is difficult to stop plaque buildup. Supplementary fluoride treatment is often prescribed.

Proper dental care for the patient taking phenytoin is based on the careful removal of food particles and the prevention of plaque buildup. The patient should avoid foods that are likely to stick in between the teeth and remain in the crevices because this sets up the kind of irritation that contributes to gum overgrowth. Many popular snacks, high in carbohydrates, are sticky and fall into this category. Patients taking phenytoin must carefully brush and floss their teeth after meals and snacks. It is necessary to reach all the tooth crevices, including those not ordinarily reached by the toothbrush. It is often inconvenient to brush the teeth after the noon meal, but dental floss can be used after the noon meal or after any snack.

Proper Brushing and Cleaning

These are sample instructions to give to patients:

1. Use a soft toothbrush and regular toothpaste
2. Hold the brush at a 45° angle to the tooth
3. Wiggle the brush slightly, beginning at the base of the teeth, and bring it up toward the top of the teeth. Do not brush sideways
4. Brush the tops of the teeth with the tip of the brush
5. Include gums in up-and-down strokes. This massages the gums, which makes them firm and resistant to irritation
6. Brush inside surface (near the tongue) and outside surface (near the cheek) of each tooth

Brushing reaches only three (inside, outside, top) of the five tooth surfaces. Use dental floss to reach the other two sides that press against neighboring teeth. Gently insert the floss between the teeth, then pull it back and forth in a sawing motion until it reaches the gums. Do this twice, once along each side of the tooth.

Water picks are another useful way of removing food particles from hard-to-reach surfaces. Plaque that does not come off with the brush may be removed with soft wood stimulators.

Vigorous regular cleaning of teeth is essential for the person taking phenytoin, but regular dental appointments are also necessary.

SELECTED READING

1. Leppik, IE. Metabolism of antiepileptic medication: newborn
to elderly. *Epilepsia* 1992;33(suppl 4):S32–S40.

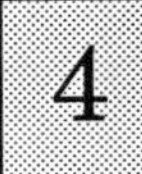

Additional Considerations In Treatment

FIRST AID FOR SEIZURES

A person having a generalized tonic-clonic seizure or a complex partial seizure should be cared for as described in the first-aid instructions given in the Appendix. The tear-out sheet may be reproduced and given to the families of epileptic patients. The diagram in the Appendix shows the proper position for placement of a patient recovering from a generalized tonic-clonic seizure. Families of patients with this type of seizure may find it useful; the tear-out copy may be reproduced and given to them.

EMERGENCY MEDICAL IDENTIFICATION

A person with epilepsy should wear or carry emergency medical identification. If a seizure occurs, the identification may reassure bystanders that the patient has a known seizure disorder and that she may not need immediate medical assistance. This could avoid an unnecessary ambulance call and fee.

Pharmacies and jewelers sell medical identification necklaces, bracelets, and charms. These usually have a standard emergency medical symbol on the front and personalized imprinting on the back.

REFERRAL TO A NEUROLOGIST

Every patient who has had a seizure does not need to be followed by a neurologist, but should be referred under certain circumstances:

1. If a referral to a comprehensive epilepsy program like MINCEP® Epilepsy Care does not require extensive travel, all referrals should be made to the epilepsy center. They will be most able to address the questions.
2. If referral to an epilepsy specialist requires extensive travel, a general neurologist should be asked to address the following problems:
   a. To confirm the diagnosis of epilepsy, to rule out psychogenic seizures, or to clarify seizure type (if proper technology is available)
   b. To evaluate unexplained abnormalities on the neurological examination
   c. Uncertainty about the cause of seizures. If the problem is definitely a seizure, could it be caused by a brain tumor, infection, or something else that needs immediate treatment?

d. Failure to achieve complete control of seizures within 3 months. Lack of control raises the question about mistakes in diagnosis or treatment. The patient may have a difficult problem that will need specialized care. The longer the patient is disabled with seizures, the harder it is to treat her.
e. Change in the type of seizure. A change in the seizure pattern raises the question of an active brain process that requires evaluation. There are other factors such as changes in the body's metabolism with drugs that may have to be evaluated.
f. An increase in the number of seizures while on an unchanged anticonvulsant level suggests than an active process is underway that should be carefully evaluated.
g. Increase in disability (mental, physical, or emotional) of the patient warrants referral to prevent further deterioration.
h. When unacceptable side effects indicate the need for alternate therapy choices
i. When initial monotherapy trial produces severe allergic reaction
j. Before embarking on combination therapy with one or more antiepileptic medicines
k. When brain MRI shows any abnormality
l. When your female patient of child-bearing potential needs advice regarding pregnancy, epilepsy, and teratogenicity of antiepileptic medicines
m. When you or your patient requires future advice regarding driving, employment restrictions, or other safety issues
n. When considering withdrawal of antiepileptic medicine
o. When the onset of seizures is associated with declining school performance, behavior disturbances, or developmental regression

3. No matter what the distance, a patient with any of the following should be referred to a comprehensive epilepsy program:
   a. Management of patients with epilepsy and magnetic resonance imaging (MRI) abnormalities of any type
   b. Consideration of surgical treatment with or without identifiable brain lesions
   c. Failure of a general neurologist to bring about complete control of seizures within 1 year
   d. Provision of expert advice regarding pregnancy or introgenicity
   e. Selection of medicine options for patients who have experienced severe drug reactions (cross-reactions are common and complicated)
   f. School learning disabilities or behavior problems
   g. Evaluation of progressive neurological decline in patients with epilepsy
   h. Consideration of the use of investigational medicines for selected patients
   i. Progressive deterioration in intellectual or social abilities or a general decline in the quality of life even with adequate seizure control

ALCOHOL AND SEIZURES

Alcohol and seizures are interconnected in a complex way. Some patients with seizures find that ingesting small amounts of alcohol worsens their seizures. These are a small minority. Most patients taking antiepileptic medicines note that their tolerance for alcohol is greatly diminished. They will get high or drunk more quickly. Newly diagnosed patients should be warned about this phenomenon.

Alcoholics have a high frequency of seizures. In most cases, these are simple withdrawal seizures due to binge drinking or to alcohol withdrawal for any reason. Alcoholics who suffer only from withdrawal seizures should *not* be treated with antiepileptic medicines. When they start drinking they forget to take their anticonvulsants and then frequently go into status epilepticus as a result of anticonvulsant withdrawal. The only way to stop the seizures is to stop the drinking.

People who abuse alcohol frequently hurt their head and develop post-traumatic seizures. Those who do so form a particularly difficult group to treat. They do need anticonvulsants to stop post-traumatic seizures, but they also tend to suffer from status epilepticus because when they start drinking they often stop taking their anticonvulsants. In addition, alcohol induces enzymes that speed up drug clearance, which shortens the half-life of many anticonvulsants. This makes seizure control much more difficult.

A seizure in an alcoholic may be the first sign of an intracranial hematoma or meningitis—don't dismiss them lightly.

CAFFEINE, STIMULANTS, STREET DRUGS, AND SEIZURES

Many people with epilepsy experience a higher frequency of seizures with large doses of caffeine. A few have this problem with smaller doses. Most people tolerate two to three cups of coffee or tea a day. Amphetamines, other stimulants, and stimulant appetite suppressants should be avoided. Theophylline, used to treat asthma, worsens seizures.

Street drugs are almost universally adulterated and misrepresented. Some contain substances that worsen a seizure disorder. All tend to interfere with the self-control needed to take charge of a seizure problem. Marijuana has no proven antiepileptic effect.

TRAUMA AND EPILEPSY

Direct physical blows to the head are a frequent cause of seizures. Often, a patient who has had a severe head injury will have a brief seizure at the time of the injury. Thus, someone who falls from a scaffold may have a seizure short-ly after hitting the ground, or a quarterback who has been sacked may have a seizure even before the opposing players have been lifted from the pileup. However, most patients do not have a seizure at the time of the injury. Many patients who have open head injuries, and a significant number of those with closed head injuries, will develop seizures later. Normally, these occur 3 months to 3 years after the injury. In rare instances, they can arise many years later.

Ordinarily, it is not difficult to treat a patient who has suffered a modest head injury and develops seizures later. Usually, all that is necessary is the prescription of ordinary doses of a common antiepileptic medicine to be taken on a regular basis (see Chapter 3). Generally, a plasma pheny-toin level of 15 to 20 μg/ml or a serum carbamazepine level of 4–6 μg/ml is satisfactory. Occasionally surgery may be needed.

Prevention of Seizures

A frequent question is whether patients with head injury should receive antiepileptic medicines to suppress or, ideal-ly, prevent the development of post-traumatic seizures. The answer is still indefinite, and medical opinion is divided. However, we must make clinical judgments nonetheless.

Patients with:

- An open brain wound (gunshot, depressed skull frac-ture)
- An injury severe enough to cause intracerebral bleeding [often diagnosed on a computerized tomography (CT) scan or by lumbar puncture and usually associated with laceration and/or contusion]
- A prolonged period of unconsciousness (>30 min) after a closed head injury
- Patients with transient focal neurological signs after a closed head injury (e.g., cranial nerve palsy) are much more likely to develop post-traumatic epilepsy.

There is good evidence that treating a patient with phenytoin at therapeutic serum levels (15–20 µg/ml) will suppress post-traumatic seizures during treatment. These patients should take anticonvulsants for 3 years after the head injury. Whether prophylactic treatment avoids development of epilepsy or merely suppresses seizures is not clear and must be subjected to further study.

LIFE-STYLE AND EPILEPSY

It is well known that emotional stress may exacerbate a seizure disorder. During periods of stress, patients with previously well-controlled epilepsy may have more seizures. If the serum drug levels are high or within the therapeutic range, management of stress may be more effective than increasing the dose of anticonvulsants.

Much has been written about diets, nutrition, trace metals, and other therapies. Regular eating habits and well-balanced meals are important in helping to regulate seizures. A few patients with rare seizure types benefit from special diets such as a high-fat ketogenic diet for absence seizures or a phenylketonuria diet for those with that disorder.

Patients may require folic acid supplements. Certain antiepileptic medicines affect folic acid levels. If folic acid deficiency is diagnosed (by a low serum level), the physician may prescribe folic acid (0.8 mg/day orally). Women of child-bearing age can help avoid neural tube defects in the fetus by taking 0.8 mg of folic acid daily (two ordinary prenatal vitamin tablets). Women taking AEDs who are planning to get pregnant should increase the dose to 4 mg/day.

Patients with only marginal seizure control often have more difficulty if they subject their bodies to sudden or extreme changes. Encourage such patients to eat adequately at regular times during the day and to sleep adequately at a regular time during the night. This will help to avoid the stresses caused by long intervals without food or sleep.

There is no need for the patient with seizures to go to bed at precisely the same hour each night. On the other hand, 3 hours of sleep each night for three nights in a row is almost guaranteed to lower the seizure threshold.

A good rule for the patient to follow is moderation in all things.

Bathing, Swimming, and Drowning

One of the more hazardous places for a patient to have a seizure is in water deep enough to cause drowning. Often the question is raised about a patient with seizures being allowed to swim. A patient whose seizures are under poor control should not swim except with immediate one-to-one supervision by a responsible adult. Other patients, with well-controlled seizure disorders, should be encouraged to swim but only if someone is with them to provide immediate assistance if needed (buddy system). Lifeguards report that it is much easier to rescue someone from a pool than from a lake or the surf.

Quite hazardous, and not generally recognized as such, is the bathtub. Patients with seizures may drown in as little as 1 to 2 inches of water if they fall face down. For this reason, some physicians advise patients with seizures to shower. Patients are more likely to lacerate their scalp if they have a seizure in the shower, but this is rarely a fatal event. Patients who are at particular risk for seizures, either because they are (a) poorly controlled, (b) being withdrawn from medicine, or (c) having their anticonvulsants changed, should not use a bathtub without someone in constant attendance who is strong enough to pull them to safety. Patients with uncontrolled seizures using a shower need be checked only occasionally.

PHYSICAL ACTIVITY AND EPILEPSY

Regular, strenuous physical activity should be encouraged for most people, including those with seizures. In general, patients with seizure disorders report that they feel better and have better seizure control when they maintain a regular exercise program. There are also examples of outstanding athletes who have epilepsy and take antiepileptic medicines.

Highly competitive individuals may find that the psychological stress of competition tends to lower their seizure threshold. However, this is an unusual circumstance that usually can be overcome with counseling and appropriate drug management.

All sports present some risk of physical injury (see Chapter 16). Even a tiddlywink can land in the eye! Take a commonsense approach to balancing the risk of a particular activity against the needs of the patient. Many factors must be considered in deciding which sports are appropriate for the individual with epilepsy. The important thing is to recognize that every case must be considered individually.

Importance of Sports to the Individual

Too often, family, friends, and society are overly protective and restrain the patient from ordinary activities. Children and adolescents engage in sports and other group activities to obtain peer group acceptance, which is important in establishing their self-image. In the balance, it may be more damaging overall to prevent the individual from participating in certain activities than to allow her to experience an accident. However, realistic limitations should be imposed if an individual has shown an interest in a high-risk activity. This problem becomes particularly acute in the case of an adolescent who has attained success in a given sport and then develops seizures. It is hard for the star quarterback of the high school team to be told that it is no longer safe for him to play football.

The situation is somewhat different in the case of professional athletes with seizures. Many of them will choose to continue in their career despite the higher risk of injury. There are professional hockey and football players and rodeo riders with seizures who knowingly accept this risk. However, they are adults who make this choice for themselves after a full explanation by their physician. Furthermore, they do not place others at risk should they have a seizure.

BIOFEEDBACK THERAPY FOR EPILEPSY

There is some evidence that biofeedback and conditioning techniques are effective in helping to control epilepsy in some patients. This type of therapy, alone, is not capable of controlling seizures. It must be used in conjunction with other medical treatments. How biofeedback works is unknown. General relaxation and stress management techniques may also be applicable in individual situations. Conditioning and deconditioning techniques for the treatment of reflex types of seizures are more specific, but also play only a limited role in overall management.

MISSED DOSES

It is common for people to miss a dose of medicine. Only rarely will missing a single dose of medicine lower the threshold enough so that the patient will have a seizure. This occurs more commonly in those drugs with a very short half-life such as valproic acid.

In general, if the patient discovers she has missed a dose, it is best to take it immediately. Most people will tolerate taking two doses of medicine at one time without serious side effects. If the patient discovers by experience that the side effects are too severe, dividing the medicine up over a period of several hours will be all that is necessary.

RHYTHMICITY IN SEIZURES

Certain patients tend to have seizures in a regular pattern, some of them just after falling asleep at night or just before awakening in the morning. Others have longer cycles, e.g., once a month, once every 45 days, or longer. We do not fully understand all the reasons for this cyclical activity, but the patient and the physician should take the seizure rhythm into consideration in planning therapy.

Menstruation and Seizures

Many women are more likely to have seizures just before or during their menses. This is a special case of seizures occurring with a rhythm. In a few cases, the seizures are related to water loading secondary to water retention, which occurs in some women just before their menses. These patients often benefit from mild salt restriction and a diuretic taken during the appropriate time of the cycle. In other cases, diuretics are of no use and the rhythmicity is related to hormonal changes.

5 Special Issues For Women With Epilepsy Genetics, Pregnancy, and Teratogenicity

PREGNANCY AND EPILEPSY

Obstetrical Considerations

Women with seizure disorders make up approximately 0.5% of all pregnant women. They present significant problems for the physician who cares for them during pregnancy and delivery. This section focuses on the major questions that are usually found in the minds of the patient and the physician. There is substantial controversy about pregnancy and epilepsy, and the opinions expressed here are derived from published reports on this subject, as well as the extensive experience of MINCEP® Epilepsy Care, Minnesota Comprehensive Epilepsy Program P.A..

A number of studies indicate that women who have epilepsy tend to have more difficulty conceiving, have a higher rate of miscarriage, and thus have a lower fertility rate. However, this is only a slight statistical difference and should be ignored in individual cases for all practical purposes.

Although eugenic laws are thankfully a thing of the past, it is wise to point out to people with epilepsy that it is better if they give some thought to heredity. Patients who come from families with a strong history of epilepsy should be advised to avoid marrying people who also come from families with a strong history of epilepsy. This is not as rare an occurrence as it might seem. Epilepsy is widely distributed in the population and the limited social opportunities available to many patients with epilepsy tend to throw them together.

When the Patient Is Seen Before Pregnancy

The woman with seizures who is not yet pregnant usually asks the physician three main questions:

1. Will antiepileptic medicines interfere with oral contraceptives or vice versa?

2. If I become pregnant, what is the risk that the child will also have seizures?
3. If I become pregnant, what is the risk that the child will be affected by antiepileptic medicines or by my epilepsy?

When the woman is already pregnant, some of the questions are moot. She usually asks:

1. What is the risk that my child will have seizures?
2. What is the risk that my antiepileptic medicines will affect the baby?
3. What are the effects of seizures occurring during pregnancy on the fetus?
4. Will my seizures become worse during pregnancy?

The obstetrician, in addition, wonders about:

1. The risk of prepartum complications
2. The risk of complications during delivery
3. The risk of postpartum complications
4. The risk of perinatal complications

Interactions Between Antiepileptic Medicines and Oral Contraceptives

A few women have reported that their seizures were markedly decreased or stopped once their menses were regulated by oral contraceptives, but the "pill" is not usually of significant help in treating seizures. The interaction of estrogens, progesterones, and antiepileptic medicines on each other's metabolism, distribution, clearance, and effectiveness is poorly understood.

There is evidence that anticonvulsants tend to decrease the effectiveness of oral contraceptives by inducing enzymes and increasing the rate of metabolism. An increase in breakthrough bleeding is a good sign that a stronger oral contraceptive is required.

If no breakthrough bleeding occurs, one can assume that the oral contraceptive is effective. Most women are not sufficiently protected from pregnancy when taking anticonvulsants and an oral contraceptive containing less than 50 mg of estrogen. The sequential formulation that provides estrogen alone for 7 days and then a progesterone/estrogen combination for 15 days has a lower progesterone content. The usual combination pill is probably a better choice and avoids the other problems associated with sequential therapy. The "mini-pill" is usually ineffective in the ordinary dosage when taken with anticonvulsants, but increasing the dosage may often produce effective contraception.

Most patients can be started on one of the low-estrogen pills that contain at least 50 mcg of estrogen. If breakthrough bleeding occurs, switch to an intermediate estrogen potency with low or intermediate progesterone content. Backup contraceptives should be used if the patient is started on a low-estrogen pill until you are satisfied that breakthrough bleeding is not occurring (see Table 5.1). I have some concern about intramuscular progesterone in patients with hard-to-control seizures. We don't have good information yet.

Many women with seizures prefer intrauterine devices (IUDs) or other contraceptive devices to the "pill." This lessens their concern about reliability, and reduces their general unhappiness at having to take so many different drugs.

Oral contraceptives rarely alter the metabolism of antiepileptic medicines. When prescribing oral contraceptives for a woman who is already taking antiepileptic medicines, it would be wise to check her serum antiepileptic medicine level to be sure that no drug interaction is occurring.

Risk of Antiepileptic Medicines Affecting the Fetus

The effect of antiepileptic medicines on the baby is a highly controversial subject that has been studied extensively in the last 20 years. The evidence favors the conclusion that

TABLE 5.1. *Choice of oral contraceptives for women taking antiepileptic medicines*

Agents listed in column A usually contain insufficient estrogen for women taking oral contraceptives. Most women taking antiepileptic medicines will find a suitable oral contraceptive option in groups B-I and B-II. A few will still have breakthrough bleeding and require a choice from column C.

<table>
<tr><td rowspan="4">P R O G E S T I N S</td><td colspan="3">Approximate Relative Oral Contraceptive Estrogen/Progestin Potency</td></tr>
<tr><td>H I G H</td><td>A-III

Demulen 1/35</td><td>B-III

Ovral</td><td>C-III

Ovulen</td></tr>
<tr><td>M E D I A T E</td><td>A-II

Lo/Ovral</td><td>B-II

Norlestrin 2.5/50</td><td>C-II

Ortho-Novum 2 mg

Norinyl 2 mg

Enovid 5 mg</td></tr>
<tr><td>L O W</td><td>A-I

Norinyl 1+50
Ortho-Novum 1/50
Ortho-Novum 1/35
Ortho-Novum 10/11
Norinyl 1+35
Ortho-Novum 7/7/7
Tri-Norinyl
Triphasil
Loestrin 1/20
Brevicon
Modicon
Ovcon-35</td><td>B-I

Norinyl 1+80
Ortho-Novum 1/80
Ovcon-50
Norlestrin 1/50</td><td>C-I

Enovid E</td></tr>
<tr><td></td><td>LOW</td><td>INTERMEDIATE</td><td>HIGH</td></tr>
</table>

ESTROGENS

From Robert J. Gumnit, M.D., reprinted with permission.

there is at least a doubling of the rate of malformations in children born to mothers who are taking antiepileptic medicines. Most of these malformations involve the cardiovascular system or the cleft palate–cleft lip syndrome, as they do in the general population. There is some suggestion that the malformations may be dose-related, but the evidence is inconclusive. Polypharmacy, especially the combination of carbamazepine, phenytoin, and valproic acid, carries a much higher risk of neural tube defects.

Recently, good evidence has been obtained that indicates that the neural tube defects associated with valproic acid (Depakene, Depakote), and carbamazepine (Tegretol) are related to folic acid deficiency. All women of child-bearing potential taking antiepileptic drugs should take a minimum of 0.4 mg and preferably 0.8 mg of folic acid a day. This is the amount found in one or two ordinary prenatal vitamin capsules. If a woman is taking antiepileptic drugs that are likely to cause a neural tube defect and is planning to get pregnant, I recommend that she begin to take 2 to 4 mg of folic acid a day before she conceives. Teratogenicity occurs during the first trimester of pregnancy, before she knows she is pregnant. The vitamin supplement must begin before she gets pregnant and continue throughout pregnancy.

A woman with a very mild seizure disorder may wish to stop taking anticonvulsants before she conceives. She must weigh the risks to herself, both physical and social, of having a seizure during pregnancy. The physician should be prepared to assist her in this decision. As a rule of thumb, she should stop the anticonvulsants at least 1 month before stopping birth control. Once the pregnancy has progressed to the middle trimester, it is generally safe to start the anticonvulsants again.

If the patient is already pregnant, there is little that can be done to decrease the risk of birth defects. By the time pregnancy is confirmed, it is too late to discuss drug withdrawals. Even so, most of the malformations that occur are uncommon (less than 6%) and are correctable. Therefore, for the woman with epilepsy who wants very much to have children, there is no reason to create undue concern or to raise the question of abortion.

Early Testing for the Possibility of Birth Defects

Most birth defects are mild, correctable, and impossible to detect before birth. Spina bifida (and similar neural tube defects), however, are detectable. At appropriate times during her pregnancy a woman taking antiepileptic drugs should have a serum alpha-fetoprotein level drawn. This is done usually at 15 to 16 weeks of gestation. Whether it is positive or negative, a high definition ultrasound examination by an experienced examiner should be performed at 18 to 19 weeks. Most women with babies with proven neural tube defects will elect to have a therapeutic abortion rather than give birth to a child who will be crippled from birth. Amniocentesis need be performed only if the alpha-fetoprotein level is elevated and the high definition ultrasound fails positively to exclude a neural tube defect.

Risk of Seizures to the Fetus

Generalized tonic-clonic seizures make severe oxygen demands on the body. Status epilepticus or prolonged seizures in the mother constitutes a medical emergency (see Chapter 8) and may affect the fetus. Fortunately, this is a relatively rare occurrence. The great majority of seizures are not accompanied by serious cardiorespiratory changes, and do not appear to affect the fetus.

Worsening of Seizures During Pregnancy

Many women with epilepsy will experience a change in seizure frequency during pregnancy. About one-third get worse, and one-third get better control. Seizures most commonly worsen during gestational ages 8 to 32 weeks. Although the mechanism is still under dispute, there is no question that serum antiepileptic medicine levels often decrease during pregnancy. Antiepileptic medicine levels (obtain unbound drug levels because of changes in protein binding during pregnancy) in pregnant women should be monitored monthly, beginning in the second trimester, and followed postpartum until the unbound levels return to normal. Antiepileptic medicine dosage should be given if needed to protect the mother. Multiple drug use increases the risk. Drug levels in the lower therapeutic range are adequate if the patient is not experiencing seizures.

Effect of Antiepileptic Medicines on Breast Milk and Breast Feeding

The amount of antiepileptic medicine secreted in breast milk is usually too small to represent a problem to the newborn. A few children have been reported to have become drowsy when breast feeding from mothers who are on high doses of ethosuximide, primidone, or phenobarbital. Unless the child develops symptoms of medication toxicity, there is no reason to avoid breast feeding.

Effect of Antiepileptic Medicines on Intelligence and Stature of the Fetus

Babies born to mothers with epilepsy tend to be smaller and of lower birth weight, but their parents are also smaller than the general population. There is no good evidence to indicate that the distribution of intelligence or head size in children born to mothers with seizures who are receiving good medical attention differs substantially from the distribution found in the parents.

Risk of Having a Child with Seizures

The risk of seizures in the general population is about 9%. Most of these seizures are single episodes and are relatively benign, that is, febrile seizures or seizure accompanying meningitis or trauma. In general, estimates of epilepsy (defined as two or more afebrile seizures separated in time) in the general population range from 1% to 2%. There is good evidence that the risk of an individual having seizures is higher if one or more close relatives have epilepsy (see the following section on genetics).

Risk of Prepartum Complications

Several studies indicate that pregnant women taking antiepileptic medicines may have an increased frequency of bleeding and placental separation. For this reason, pregnant women with seizures should be followed closely by an obstetrician. Vitamin K can be given one month before labor, especially to patients on phenobarbital.

Risk of Complications During Delivery

If the woman has no coagulation problems, complications during delivery do not appear to be significantly increased. Antiepileptic medicines can affect the mother's vitamin K-dependent clotting mechanisms. These should be checked before delivery.

Risk of Perinatal Complications to the Fetus

Some infants born to mothers taking antiepileptic medicines have a vitamin K-deficiency-type of bleeding diathesis. The administration of additional vitamin K to the mother 3 weeks before delivery and to the fetus at delivery is appropriate.

Infants do not appear to be particularly sedated from maternal antiepileptic medicines. There have been a few reports of withdrawal symptoms in the child after delivery, but sedation does not appear to be a significant complication.

Managing the Mother Through Pregnancy

With all these forces at work, it is clear that a woman who is taking antiepileptic medicines needs very careful attention before getting pregnant, during pregnancy and delivery, and in the first 6 to 12 weeks after delivery. More than 90% of the time everything goes well without any difficulties. However, a pregnant woman taking antiepileptic medicines should be seen somewhat more frequently by her obstetrician during the last trimester and will require close attention to her antiepileptic blood levels, especially during the last trimester. It may be necessary to increase the dose of the antiepileptic medications, as the levels often fall just before delivery. After delivery, when the liver returns to normal, it will be necessary to reduce the dose. Some women will experience toxicity from the medicines and this should be avoided if possible, especially if she is breast feeding.

Breast Feeding

A woman who is taking antiepileptic medicines need not be concerned about breast feeding her baby. The benefits of breast feeding far outweigh the slight risk of the baby getting sick from antiepileptic medicines that the mother is taking. The amount of antiepileptic medicine that the baby receives from mother's milk is generally small and does not create any clinical problems. On rare occasions the baby may be sedated, appear to be sleepy, and feed poorly as the result of high levels of antiepileptic medicines in the mother's milk. In this case, it may be wise to switch partially or wholly to formula. Feeding difficulties and decreased weight gain have been proved only in those mothers taking phenobarbital and primidone (Mysoline), and it is unusual even with these medicines.

Instructions for the Mother

Having a baby may bring a lot of joy; it also brings a lot of stress. Lack of sleep, hormonal changes, and the extra work and anxiety associated with a new baby in the house makes things worse. Mothers need to take time to rest. If their sleep has been disturbed during the night they will need a nap. Fathers should help out with nighttime feedings and baby care; this not only helps the mother but also helps create a closer bond between father and baby.

Are Seizures a Risk to the Baby?

There have been remarkably few confirmed events in which a baby was harmed by a mother having seizures. There is no reason to discourage nearly all women with epilepsy from having children because they might harm the baby. There are, however, some sensible precautions. If the mother has frequent seizures, someone else should bathe the baby, because drowning is a particular risk. If she has seizures in which she might drop the baby or fall to the floor, the baby can be changed or fed sitting on the floor. If the baby is on a changing table, strap the baby securely.

One of the bigger risks is holding the baby while cooking. Like the risk for drowning, the risk for burns is particularly great under these circumstances. It is best to leave the baby in a seat nearby or in a playpen.

Once the baby begins to toddle and walk, the precautions need to be increased. Whether or not the mother has seizures, a house needs to be made child-proof. Irons and ironing boards should not be left out; electrical plugs should have covers; drawers and cupboards should have child-proof latches.

If the mother has seizures or periods of confusion, special precautions should be taken. Doors to the kitchen, bathroom, and the outside should be locked or otherwise fixed so that the baby cannot let himself out but help can come in. Not only should the usual precautions of keeping soaps, polishes, and bleaches away from the child be observed, but the mother must be careful that her antiepileptic medicines are not within reach.

GENETIC FACTORS IN SEIZURES

Genetic Principles

Understanding genetic principles can help the physician treat patients with seizures. Progress is being made in understanding the mechanisms involved and the implications for diagnosis and treatment of epilepsy.

A small proportion of cases of seizures (perhaps less than 5%) result from a chromosome anomaly or a Mendelian genetic trait. If the seizure patient shows a complex set of malformations, the possibility of a chromosome disorder should be investigated. There are more than 100 different Mendelian traits (such as tuberous sclerosis) that increase the risk of seizures. One-third of these lead to mental retardation in addition to seizures.

The remaining cases of epilepsy arise from a combination of genetic and environmental factors, much as in other common medical problems. In the case of epilepsy, the genetic factors are largely at work in the patient's basic threshold for seizures. It is the interaction of this genetically determined threshold with the immediate precipitating cause that determines whether or not a seizure actually occurs. For example, not all infants who develop a fever will develop febrile seizures. Some will have one at 102°F; others, at 105°F; and others, not at all. Similarly, most people do not develop seizures in response to discotheque lights in the 10- to 15-Hz range, but those with a genetic predisposition to photically induced epilepsy may.

Family History of Seizures

A history of seizures in a parent of the epileptic patient should be considered carefully, even if the seizures in the patient appear to have arisen from straightforward, identifiable causes. When a parent is affected, the risk to siblings is as high for a patient with a single symptomatic seizure as for a patient with recurrent idiopathic seizures. A family history of epilepsy may also be relevant for patients who have had a single seizure. The recurrence rate appears to be higher among those with a history of seizures in a parent or sibling.

Genetic Counseling—Population at Risk

The physician should be prepared to offer genetic counseling or to refer the patient to an appropriate center. The patient usually asks about the likelihood of siblings or children of the patient developing seizures. About 2% of persons in the general population develop recurring seizures by age 40 years, but this risk is increased to 4% to 5% for siblings and children of affected persons. The risk is higher (in the range of 6–8%) if any of the following is observed:

- Early (childhood or teenage) seizure onset in the patient
- A parent who has seizures (less risk if only the father has seizures)
- A sibling who has seizures
- A spike-and-wave pattern in the patient's EEG

SELECTED READINGS

1. Dam M, Christiansen J, Munck O, Mygind KJ. Antiepileptic drugs: metabolism in pregnancy. *Clin Pharmacokinetics* 1979;4:53–62.
2. Ramsay RE, Strauss RG, Wilder BJ, Willmore LJ. Status epilepticus in pregnancy: effect of phenytoin malabsorption on seizure control. *Neurology* 1978;28:85–89.
3. Wilson JT, Brown RD, Cherek BR, et al. Drug excretion in human breast milk: principles, pharmacokinetics and projected consequences. *Clin Pharmacokinetics* 1980;5:1–66.
4. Battino D, Avanzini G, Bossi L, et al. Monitoring of antiepileptic plasma levels during pregnancy and puerperium. In: *Epilepsy, pregnancy, and the child*. New York: Raven Press, 1982:147–154.
5. Anderson VE, Rich SS, Hauser WA, Wilcox KJ. Family studies of epilepsy. In: Anderson VE, Hauser WA, Leppik IE, Nobles JL, Rich SS, eds. *Genetic strategies in epilepsy research. Epilepsy Research*. Amsterdam: Elsevier; 1991(suppl 4):89–103.
6. Hauser WA, Annegers JF. Risk factors for epilepsy. In: Anderson VE, Hauser WA, Leppik IE, Nobles JL, Rich SS, eds. *Genetic strategies in epilepsy research. Epilepsy Research*. Amsterdam: Elsevier; 1991(suppl 4):45–51.

Treatment Of Children With Epilepsy

6

EARLY INTERVENTION

Seizures are not good for the brain. Dependency and social isolation are not good for the soul. Physicians and parents should strive to bring seizures under control at the earliest opportunity. This will help minimize dependency and social isolation. Uncontrolled seizures when the adolescent is learning independence, job skills, dating, and driving can warp an entire life. Our treatment aims must be:

- No seizures
- No side effects

Early referral of patients with persistent seizures to a specialized epilepsy center should be encouraged.

DIFFERENTIAL DIAGNOSIS

One of the major problems in the differential diagnosis of seizures in young children is distinguishing between febrile seizures, breath-holding spells, and epilepsy. Key differentiating points are shown in Table 6.1. The differential diagnosis of seizures in children includes many different "behaviors" that can resemble epileptic seizure activity. These phenomena can be classified according to whether they occur in relation to the waking or sleep states. For example, children with "night terrors" or a newborn baby in "rapid eye movement" sleep with frequent "jerky" eye movements and irregular breathing can appear to be having seizures. The toddler with "breath-holding spells" or the adolescent with apparently unprovoked "rage attacks" are often referred to an epilepsy center for evaluation of their suspected seizures.

ABSENCE AND COMPLEX PARTIAL SEIZURES

Neonatal seizures may be encountered in very young infants, but once a child has gone beyond the first year of life,

TABLE 6.1 *Significant factors in differential diagnosis of seizures in children*

	Febrile seizures	Breath-holding spells	Epilepsy
History	Only with fever	Provoked by pain, anger, frustration	Usually unpredictable
Age	6 mo–5 yr	6 mo–4 yr	Any age
EEG	Normal when afebrile	Normal; may have an abnormal EKG/EEG with ocular compression	Often interictal paroxysmal activity
Treatment	Optional, with valproic acid or carbamazepine	Accurate diagnosis; parental counse ing	Essential with appropriate AEM

EKG, electrocardiogram; EEG, electroencephalogram; AEM, antiepileptic medicine.

the likelihood of seizures beginning in the absence of a clear-cut precipitating event such as meningitis is relatively small until age 3 years. Absence seizures or similar types of generalized spells generally start between the ages of 4 and 10 years. Although this is the ordinary age for such seizures to begin, simple, uncomplicated absence seizures are not common. However, when the electroencephalogram (EEG) is typical (bilaterally synchronous and symmetrical 3/sec spikes and waves, maximal over F_1 and F_2), and especially if there is a family history of seizures or a response to hyperventilation, the physician can be comfortable in treating the child with ethosuximide or, if that fails, valproic acid.

Most children who have seizures in preadolescence, however, suffer from the same types of partial seizures that affect adults. These children may have simple or complex partial seizures. If they have had severe diffuse brain damage, mixed seizures of multifocal origin may be seen. This particular group of patients may be especially hard to treat. The basic rules still apply. If the medical history and EEG are typical and the child responds promptly to standard doses of an anticonvulsant, the family physician will rarely encounter difficulty in treatment. If the seizures do not respond to treatment, or if the clinical situation is poorly understood, the child should be referred to a pediatric neurologist. Once the situation is understood and the seizures controlled, continuing care can frequently be resumed by the family physician.

As the child gains weight, the amount of drug needed for seizure control will increase because more drug is needed for distribution in the growing body. A careful comparison of recommended dosages between adults and children indicates that the rules of thumb applicable to adults may not be appropriate in the case of children.

EEG in Childhood Seizures

Competent EEGs are mandatory to treat seizures properly. Many neurologists have little experience interpreting EEGs in young children. False diagnoses of epilepsy are made too frequently. Often, relatively benign findings, for example, unusual arousal patterns, Rolandic small sharp spikes, or Rolandic epilepsy, are misinterpreted. Properly diagnosing and treating epilepsy in infants, toddlers, and young children is usually difficult. No physician should be ashamed or hesitate to ask for help from a pediatric neurologist or an epilepsy center.

FEBRILE SEIZURES

Generalized tonic-clonic seizures in young children who have a high fever, generally between the ages of 1 and 4 years, are common. Three percent of the cases of nonrecurrent seizures in Rochester, Minnesota, were of this type. In general, these seizures are benign and do not require treatment. The appearance of seizures with a high fever is an expression of a genetically determined threshold for seizures that is lower than the average. If the seizure is brief, treating the fever with acetominophen and cool water baths is all that is necessary. When the seizures are repeated frequently, many physicians elect to treat with antiepileptic medicines, which is particularly appropriate if any of the seizures have been prolonged. Prolonged seizures, even with maintenance of good respiration, may cause further brain damage. In fact, some cases of complex partial seizures are thought to arise from brain damage produced by febrile seizures. Prolonged seizures can be treated at home by the parents on an episodic basis with oral Ativan or rectal Valium.

Traditionally, physicians prescribed prophylactic phenobarbital in small doses. This is a relatively safe and effective choice of drugs, but there is no question that phenobarbital, even in low doses, will produce drowsiness in some children and slow learning in many children, and cause hyperactivity in others, especially those with underlying brain damage. Other drugs that may be used are valproic acid, which has the serious risk of liver toxicity in infants, and carbamazepine, which has a higher incidence of blood dyscrasias than does phenobarbital.

Children with febrile seizures who have clinical or EEG evidence of focal neurological damage suffer from both lowered seizure threshold with fever and brain damage. They do not belong to the group of patients with simple, benign febrile seizures, and probably should be treated.

ANTIEPILEPTIC MEDICINES COMMONLY USED FOR CHILDREN

This information serves as a broad guideline for the use of anticonvulsants in children. The proper dosage for each patient depends on many factors, including age, weight, severity of the epileptogenic process, associated central nervous system disease, and gastrointestinal, hepatic, or renal function. The drugs are listed alphabetically by generic name.

Carbamazepine (Tegretol)

Indications: Complex partial seizures, generalized tonic-clonic seizures, partial seizures secondarily generalized, elementary partial seizures
Average daily dose: 10 to 30 mg/kg
Formulation: 200 mg tablets, 100 mg chewable tablets, suspension 100 mg/5 ml
Metabolism: Hepatic conversion to epoxide and other metabolites
Serum half-life: 12 ± 6 hr
Time to achieve steady state: 2 to 4 days
Effective blood level: >4 μg/ml
Toxic level (dose-related side effects): >13 μg/ml

Ethosuximide (Zarontin)

Indications: Absence seizures
Average daily dose: 20 to 40 mg/kg
Formulation: 250 mg capsules (soft gel capsules can be frozen and sliced for fractional doses); 250 mg/5 ml syrup
Metabolism: Hepatic
Serum half-life: 30 ± 6 hr
Time to achieve steady state: 5 to 10 days
Effective blood level: >40 μg/ml
Toxic level (dose-related side effects): >150 μg/ml
Note: Gastric irritation is a common side effect at therapeutic levels (medication should be taken with meals); hiccups are common at higher levels

Felbamate (Felbatol)

Indications: Complex partial seizures, drop attacks, tonic-clonic, and atypical absence seizures in Lennox-Gasteux syndrome
Contraindications: None

Average daily dose: 1,200 to 3,600 mg/day or more if necessary

Formulation: Tablets of 400 and 600 mg, suspension 600 mg/5 ml

Metabolism: Hydroxylation and conjugation in the liver

Serum half-life: 14 hr

Time to achieve steady state: 3 days

Effective blood level: Not known, tentatively greater than 50 μg/ml

Toxic level (dose-related side effects): Not known

Common side effects: Insomnia, weight loss, decreased appetite, dizziness, fatigue. A rash may be seen if the patient is also taking Depakote.

On August 1, 1994 the FDA reported that adults taking Felbatol had and incidence of aplastic anemia 20-50 times higher than the gernal population. No children were reported with the disorder by August 8, 1994. Physicians should reserve Felbatol for those children whose seizures present a serious problem and who have not responded to safer AED's.

Phenobarbital

Indications: Generalized tonic-clonic seizures, elementary partial seizures, partial seizures secondarily generalized

Contraindications: Absence seizures, atypical absence seizures, drop attacks

Average daily dose: 3 to 8 mg/kg

Formulation: 8 mg, 15 mg, 30 mg, 60 mg, and 100 mg tablets, elixir 400 mg/100 ml

Metabolism: Hydroxylated by the liver, but a significant amount is excreted unchanged by the kidneys

Serum half-life: 96 ± 12 hr

Time to achieve steady state: 14 to 21 days

Effective blood level: >20 μg/ml

Toxic level (dose-related side effects): >40 μg/ml

Common side effects: Hyperactivity, sedation, personality changes, and learning difficulties are common side effects at therapeutic levels. Avoid the use of phenobarbital if possible.

Phenytoin (Dilantin)

Indications: Generalized tonic-clonic seizures, elementary partial seizures, complex partial seizures, partial seizures secondarily generalized
Average daily dose: 3 to 8 mg/kg
Formulation: 30 mg and 100 mg capsules; 50 mg chewable tablets, scored (bioavailability different from capsules); suspension (unreliable, not recommended for routine use) 125 mg/5 ml, 30 mg/5 ml
Metabolism: Hydroxylated by liver (small increases in dose may result in large increases in plasma level)
Serum half-life: 24 ± 12 hr
Time to achieve steady state: 5 to 10 days
Effective blood level: >10 μg/ml
Toxic level (dose-related side effects): >20 μg/ml
Common side effects: Gingival hypertrophy, hirsutism, and coarsening of features are potential side effects at therapeutic levels. Be prepared to change to another antiepileptic drug in adolescence if severe acne or hirsutism develop. Gingival hypertrophy can be avoided by proper dental hygiene.

Primidone (Mysoline)

Indications: Generalized tonic-clonic seizures, elementary partial seizures, complex partial seizures, partial seizures secondarily generalized
Average daily dose: 10 to 25 mg/kg
Formulation: 50 mg and 250 mg tablets, scored; suspension 250 mg/5 ml
Metabolism: Hepatic conversion to phenobarbital and phenylethylmalonamide

Serum half-life: 12 ± 6 hr (96 ± 12 hr for phenobarbital)
Time to achieve steady state: 4 to 7 days (14–21 days for phenobarbital)
Effective blood level: >5 μg/ml
Toxic level (dose-related side effects): >15 μg/ml of primidone; >40 μg/ml of phenobarbital
Common side effects: Sedation and hyperactivity are common side effects at therapeutic levels. Dizziness, ataxia, and nausea may occur unless initial dosage is low (1–2 mg/kg) and gradually increased

Valproic Acid (Depakene/Depakote)

Indications: Absence seizures, myoclonic seizures, generalized tonic-clonic seizures, complex partial seizures
Average daily dose: 750 to 2,000 mg (20–60 mg/kg), divided into three or more doses
Formulation: Depakene 250 mg capsules; 250 mg/5 ml syrup. Depakote 125, 250, 500 mg tablets, 125 mg "sprinkles"
Metabolism: Hepatic
Serum half-life: 10 ± 6 hr
Time to achieve steady state: 2 to 4 days
Effective blood level: >50 μg/ml
Toxic level (dose-related side effects): >100 μg/ml
Common side effects: Gastric irritation is a common side effect at therapeutic levels (medication should be taken with meals). Dosage of phenobarbital and related drugs should be reduced by one-third when valproic acid is added to avoid rapid increase in plasma barbiturate levels.

THE PHYSICIAN, THE CHILD WITH EPILEPSY, AND THE SCHOOL

It is important that the parents, physician, school personnel, and child all communicate and operate from the same set of facts. Most children with epilepsy can remain in a regular classroom because they do not differ from ordinary students in intelligence, ability, or achievement. Some

children with epilepsy may need special education programs, ordinarily for the same reasons that children without epilepsy may need special programs. Each child must
be considered as an individual.

Epilepsy involves adjustments on the part of the child
and the family. Those aspects of the disorder that cannot be
altered, no matter how well they are understood, must be
lived with. School personnel can help the child learn to live
well with epilepsy by recognizing and understanding how
the disorder may affect the individual child.

Most children with epilepsy have to learn to live with the
possibility of lifelong seizures. Although seizures in most children are well controlled with medication, and many children
may eventually be able to stop taking antiepileptic medicines,
none should look forward to a cure. This must be accepted
without pity by both the child and the school. Teachers should
never expect less from a child with epilepsy, in class work or
behavior, simply because she has seizures.

The impairment of most chronic disorders is continuous,
but seizures occur episodically. No child, family, teacher, or
physician can predict when a seizure will occur. This fact
makes it harder to adjust to epilepsy. A child whose seizures
are well controlled is usually fearful of having another seizure.
Anxiety will be lessened if the child can expect proper care
during the seizure and continued acceptance afterward.

The fact that the cause of epilepsy is unknown, and the
knowledge that the duration of treatment with antiepileptic
medicines is indefinite, creates uncertainty for both the
child and the family. Ordinarily, the physician will not
know the cause of a child's epilepsy, but this does not mean
a worse prognosis or a lesser chance of medical control.
Teachers may help relieve the anxiety provoked by the
uncertainty by providing support to the family and the
child. Children and their families worry about the side
effects of the antiepileptic medicines, and that may add
another element of uncertainty. The overwhelming majority of children have minimal or no side effects. Teachers

should encourage children and parents to ask their physicians directly should they have questions about side effects of the medications.

Social Problems

Throughout history, epilepsy has been regarded differently in different societies. In some cultures, the patient with seizures was thought to have divine powers; in others, the patient was driven away or placed in an institution. Even today, many people think epilepsy causes mental illness or retardation. A social stigma surrounds epilepsy that may affect the child and her family to varying degrees.

One of our most highly prized qualities is self-control. Most of us want to feel and appear in control of ourselves, and society demands that we do so. During a seizure, all semblance of self-control may be lost, even of the bowel and bladder. This is frightening to most observers, as well as to the person with seizures.

No one is completely independent, no matter how highly we prize independence, but the child with epilepsy may be taught to be unnecessarily dependent. Certainly, the necessity for daily medication, frequent visits to the physician, and restrictions in employment and driving create serious stresses. The child with epilepsy does not normally think of herself as sick and, except during the seizure, she is often as healthy as anyone else. It is important not to encourage an attitude of sickness.

The natural tendency of parents and teachers is to be overprotective of the child with epilepsy. This is understandable, but overprotection is destructive because the child is not allowed to learn from mistakes and experience. Overprotection often leads to expectations of preferential treatment. Children with epilepsy must learn to be responsible for the management of their own problems. Taking medication and making decisions about physical and other restrictions must gradually become the responsibility of the child.

Exercise is important to everyone, especially those with seizures. Every child, even those with seizures, should be encouraged to participate actively in sports and exercise. If certain activities must be restricted because of poor seizure control, substitute exercise must be found. Children whose seizures are well controlled with medication can participate in all the activities of their classmates (see Chapter 5).

Driving

Students of eligible age should be encouraged to take the classroom part of driver's training, even if their seizures are poorly controlled. Seizure control should be actively pursued, and when the child becomes eligible for a license, insurance premiums will be lower because of the training. Because much of driver's education pertains to general and pedestrian safety, it is beneficial to nondrivers as well.

Medication During School Hours

It is often inconvenient and embarrassing for a child to take antiepileptic medicines at school. Many schools have an illicit drug problem and prohibit students from carrying even prescribed medication. Medications usually have to be administered by the school nurse. Parents should consult the physician about creating a dosage schedule that can avoid school hours. Many antiepileptic medicines can be given on a twice-a-day schedule without difficulty. Nearly all patients can go from 8 a.m. until 4 p.m. without taking medication, especially if the last dose of the day is taken in the evening.

Information to the School

Teachers need information from the family and physicians if they are to assist in caring for the child with seizures. This information is best prepared by the family and physician working together. A form that has been found helpful in transmitting this information is found in the Appendix. The tear-out copy may be reproduced and adapted for use.

Information From the School

The family and the physician need information from the school. Upon request, teachers should be expected to provide information about:

- Recorded observation of all seizures (see anecdotal record in Appendix; the tear-out form may be copied and given to the teacher)
- Changes in child's behavior that may indicate medication side effects (lethargy, blurred vision, difficulty seeing the blackboard)
- Unexplained changes in school performance
- Increase in frequency or severity of seizures
- Behavioral and/or social problems that may require referral for counseling

SELECTED READINGS

1. Aicardi J. *Epilepsy in children*. New York: Raven Press, 1986.
2. Aicardi J. *Diseases of the nervous system in childhood, Chapters 16, 17, and 30*. London: Mac Keith Press.
3. Holmes GL. Diagnosis and management of seizures in children. *Major problems in clinical pediatrics,* vol. 30. Philadelphia: W.B. Saunders, 1987.
4. Roger J, Dravet C, Bureau M, Dreifuss FE, Wolf P. *Epileptic syndromes in infancy, childhood and adolescence*. London: John Libbey, Eurotext, 1985.

Treatment Of Infants With Seizures

7

GUIDELINES FOR TREATING NEONATAL SEIZURES

Seizures in the first month of life take many forms. Generalized tonic-clonic movements are the least common. It is more common to see:

- Focal tonic or clonic movements of a single extremity
- Opisthotonic posturing
- Intermittent apneic episodes with cyanosis and bradycardia
- Facial grimacing
- Sudden loss of muscle tone
- Myoclonic spasms
- Bicycling movements

The form the seizures take is related to the functional capacity of the newborn's brain and not to the etiology of the seizure.

Seizures as Secondary Abnormality

All seizures in the neonatal period must be assumed to be secondary to a serious underlying abnormality of central nervous system function. Failure to treat certain of these underlying abnormalities in a timely fashion can lead to permanent neurological sequelae or death. All neonatal seizures should be considered diagnostic and therapeutic emergencies.

Etiology

The most common identifiable causes of neonatal seizures are:

- Hypoglycemia (treatable)
- Hypocalcemia (treatable)
- Infection (treatable)
- Hypomagnesemia (treatable)
- Fetal hypoxia
- Intracranial hemorrhage
- Congenital anomalies
- Postmaturity
- Intrauterine growth retardation

Less common but specific causes include:

- Inborn errors of metabolism (particularly aminoacidopathies)
- Abnormalities of short-chain fatty acid metabolism
- Disorders of the urea cycle
- Other rare disorders

Emergency Diagnosis

Minimal emergency diagnostic procedures essential to the key diagnosis include:

- Lumbar puncture
- Blood culture
- Blood glucose
- Serum calcium
- Serum magnesium
- Serum electrolytes
- Blood urea nitrogen

Also, obtain blood titers for toxoplasmosis, rubella, cytomegalovirus, Herpes simplex, and syphilis. Magnetic resonance imaging (MRI) of the head should be performed.

Emergency Treatment

The following is a guide for treating the full-term newborn. If you have a premature newborn with repetitive seizures, call a neonatal intensive care center for advice *immediately*.

1. Start treatment for certain causes of neonatal seizures even before laboratory results are available. Support respiration if necessary.
   a. Begin appropriate administration of antibiotics for possible sepsis and meningitis.
   b. Administer 5 to 10 ml of a 20% to 30% glucose solution (0.5–1 mg/kg i.v.) for possible hypoglycemia, with electrocardiogram (EKG) monitoring.
2. If seizures do not stop within 5 min, slowly administer 2 to 6 ml of 2.5% to 5% calcium gluconate (20–120 mg/kg i.v.), with EKG monitoring.
3. If seizures do not stop in another 5 min, then slowly administer 2 to 6 ml of 2% to 3% magnesium sulphate (40–180 mg i.v.). Administer 16 to 72 mg/kg and monitor EKG for bradycardia.
4. If seizures continue, administer pyridoxine (50 mg i.v.), and observe for 3 min.
5. If seizures continue after these specific treatments have been given, then administer phenobarbital, currently the drug of choice for neonatal seizures. An appropriate load-

ing dose is 20 mg/kg. This produces a serum level of approximately 20 to 25 µg/ml between 30 min and 6 hr after an i.v. dose. (Intramuscular administration is also effective.) Sedation and central nervous system depression have not been a problem with this dose. Additional doses or maintenance doses will not be needed for several days. Their need should be determined by the serum phenobarbital levels.

6. If seizures do not stop, give an additional 10 mg/kg of phenobarbital after 4 to 6 hr. Serum levels should then be checked as described above.
7. If an adequate phenobarbital loading dose does not lead to seizure control, give a loading dose of phenytoin 20 mg/kg i.v. Phenytoin must be given intravenously because intramuscular absorption is unreliable. Do not administer phenytoin orally because it is irregularly absorbed in the neonate. If seizures continue or the diagnosis is still in doubt after initial diagnostic and therapeutic efforts, the infant should be referred to a pediatric neurologist or intensivist. Early referral is desirable.

MORTALITY AND MORBIDITY

The seriousness of neonatal seizures cannot be overemphasized. The mortality rate is about 20%, and the late morbidity rate is about 50%. Suboptimal management of these seizures may cause lifelong retardation with sensorimotor handicaps.

8 Status Epilepticus

A MEDICAL EMERGENCY

Convulsive status epilepticus is a medical emergency. Left untreated, many patients will die. With improper treatment, many may suffer serious brain damage and long-term disability. Since status epilepticus, like all seizures, is a symptom, the prognosis varies with the etiology of the seizures. Status epilepticus secondary to severe hypoxic brain damage is extremely resistant to therapy and will often lead to death. Status epilepticus is a grave symptom when associated with brain infection or trauma; however, prompt treatment of the infection or the hematoma will often cure the patient.

In about half the cases of status epilepticus this event was the patient's first seizure. Any kind of seizure may be manifested by status epilepticus, but the life-threatening cases are associated with generalized convulsive movements. Although appropriate and timely therapy can reduce death and injury, the ultimate prognosis is most closely related to the etiology. About 3% of children and 10% of adults will die from convulsive status epilepticus *per se* but overall 8% of children and about 30% of adults with convulsive status epilepticus will die, in large part because of the associated underlying conditions.

Status epilepticus can be defined as more than 30 min of continuous partial seizure activity or two or more generalized seizures in a row without full recovery of consciousness between seizures. Although repeated partial seizures, such as continuous focal motor convulsions or continuous nonconvulsive complex partial seizures producing a "twilight state" from epilepsy, are not rare, they are nowhere near as common and certainly nowhere near as dangerous as repeated generalized convulsive seizures with persistent postictal depression of neurological function between the seizures. Respiratory depression and cardiovascular collapse are the most urgent concerns.

CAUSES OF STATUS EPILEPTICUS

The most common cause of status epilepticus is a sudden drop in serum levels of antiepileptic medicines caused by failure to take the medication or by increased clearance associated with intercurrent illness. Withdrawal of antiepileptic medicines may occur because:

- The patient may run out of medicine and fail to refill the prescriptions
- The patient may take the medicine only sporadically
- The patient may lose the medicine and not obtain another supply
- The patient may decide that antiepileptic medicines are no longer needed
- The patient may misunderstand the physician's instructions
- The physician may decide that there is no longer any need for antiepileptic medicines and instruct the patient to stop or decrease the dose too abruptly

Status epilepticus also occurs for unknown reasons in patients with epilepsy who have not altered their drug intake. Fever and systemic infections can increase clearance and lower serum levels of the drugs and thus bring about status epilepticus. Substitute "generic" drugs may have lower bioavailability. Status epilepticus can also be caused by acute central nervous system disorders such as hypoxia, eclampsia, hypoglycemia, encephalitis, meningitis, head injury, subarachnoid hemorrhage, stroke, metabolic encephalopathy, and toxicity from cocaine, angel dust, theophylline, and other poisons. Status epilepticus from these causes is often difficult to control.

Status epilepticus may result from the sudden cessation of depressant drugs such as barbiturates or benzodiazepines. Almost any sleeping pill will cause seizures if the patient has been taking large doses for a long time and then suddenly stops. Status epilepticus from this cause is usually easily treated with phenytoin or almost any other antiepileptic medicine if the problem is recognized. Examine the urine for toxic metabolites. Careful questioning of the family may be helpful in making the diagnosis.

Status epilepticus occurs in about 20% of patients experiencing seizures for the first time. This means that except in the case of a patient who is well known to the physician, and who has a history of stopping antiepileptic medicines, the physician must be prepared to undertake an emergency evaluation. First, stop the seizures and restore adequate respiration and circulation. Once the major motor seizures have been stopped, take time to identify the cause of the seizures. Consider direct infections of the nervous system, systemic infections of the body, toxin exposure, and metabolic disturbances. Subarachnoid hemorrhage, not immediately apparent trauma, nonhemorrhagic vascular insults, tumors, subdural hematomas, and degenerative diseases are other possible causes. Infants and elderly patients with status epilepticus require vigorous efforts to find a symptomatic etiology.

GENERAL PRINCIPLES OF TREATMENT

The aim of treatment is to terminate seizure activity rapidly with minimal depression of consciousness and cardiopulmonary function. First provide an adequate airway and respiratory support, and obtain access to a good vein. Monitor blood pressure, electrocardiogram (EKG), respiration, and temperature. Then, while beginning drug treatment, it is necessary to rule out certain causes of the status epilepticus. If a patient is in status owing to hyponatremia, hypoglycemia, or acute metabolic disturbance, the seizures will not stop until this problem is corrected. Obtain specimens for the following baseline determinations:

- Serum sodium
- Potassium

- Calcium
- Chloride
- Glucose
- Carbon dioxide
- Blood urea nitrogen
- Antiepileptic medicine levels

An intravenous injection of 50% glucose may be given before antiepileptic medicines are used. If hypoglycemia is the cause of status epilepticus, the glucose injection will stop the seizures. Be sure to draw a blood sample for serum glucose determination before giving the injection.

ADULTS AND STATUS EPILEPTICUS

Types of Status Epilepticus in Adults

Generalized status epilepticus is a state of continuous or repetitive generalized tonic-clonic seizures, without an intervening return of consciousness. Under these conditions, the patient is usually in respiratory distress. If respiration is not impaired, consider the possibility of nonepileptic psychogenic seizures.

Most tonic-clonic seizures are self-limited, of short duration (55 sec), and do not require emergency treatment with drugs. A tonic-clonic seizure lasting longer than 2 min should alert the physician to the possible need for medical treatment of status epilepticus and such treatment should be initiated immediately.

It is possible to have continuous absence seizures or continuous simple or complex partial seizures (old terms: continuous petit mal or psychomotor seizures). Although medical attention is needed with these types of status epilepticus, they are not life-threatening. Status epilepticus with generalized tonic-clonic seizures is life-threatening, with the patient at severe cardiorespiratory risk.

There is good evidence from animal experiments that continuous seizures can produce brain damage, even if respiration is adequately maintained. The problem is compounded if the patient is hypoxic and acidotic. All the steps outlined below can be completed within 5 to 10 min. If 15 min have passed and the seizures persist, anesthetize and intubate the patient and call a consultant.

Guidelines for Treatment of Status Epilepticus in Adults

1. Secure an unobstructed airway. Assist respiration as necessary. Give supplemental oxygen as necessary.
2 Get a good i.v. going and maintain blood pressure.
3. Monitor EKG, respiration, blood pressure, body temperature. Do not overhydrate.
4. Diagnose the condition and its cause.
5. Measure antiepileptic medicine levels in patients with known seizures.
6. Give initial doses of drugs intravenously.
7. Give adequate doses of medications from the start.
8. Do not hesitate to reconsider your working diagnosis of the cause of the status epilepticus if seizures continue.
9. Do not switch from the parenteral to the oral route of drug administration until seizures have stopped.
10. Once status epilepticus is controlled, consider maintenance therapy.
11. Avoid short-acting barbiturates because they work only by anesthetizing the patient.

Maintain respiratory function (intubate as necessary). Carefully watch cardiac status. Obtain a blood specimen and determine baseline values for blood levels of sodium, potassium, calcium, chloride, glucose, carbon dioxide, urea nitrogen, and antiepileptic medicines. Using the same vena puncture through which the blood specimen was obtained, start an i.v. line immediately. Administer one ampule of 50% glucose injection (25 g of glucose). If there is even the slightest question of alcohol abuse, thiamine should be given (100 mg i.v.), injected with the glucose, to avoid precipitating a Wernicke's encephalopathy. Other water-soluble vitamins, especially pyridoxine, may be required.

If respiratory function is not in jeopardy, and the patient's color is acceptable, a minute or two can be taken at this point to do brief neurological and physical examinations to rule out acute structural causes of the seizure disturbance. This may be difficult because pupil reactivity, focal motor seizure activity, or Todd's paralysis can cause confusion. Findings of a hemotympanum, Battle's sign, raccoon sign, a nonfluctuating, persistently dilated pupil that is unreactive to light, or persistent lateralized weakness without fluctuation over several minutes should all be considered signs of a possible significant, acute structural etiology (e.g., trauma or tumor). History should be obtained from all possible sources. If, at any point, respiratory or cardiac function appears in jeopardy, or the generalized motor seizures have persisted too long, i.v. administration of antiepileptic medicines should begin.

DRUG THERAPY FOR STATUS EPILEPTICUS IN ADULTS

Lorazepam

Lorazepam (Ativan) is (for me) the drug of choice in the treatment of status. It is relatively safe, enters the brain rapidly, and has a prolonged antiepileptic effect. It is slightly faster when administered intravenously, but can be given intramuscularly (i.m.). For a full-sized adult give 3 to 4 mg initially, over a 2- to 4-min period in an attempt to terminate seizures rapidly. This may be repeated every 15 min until a total of 8 to 10 mg has been administered. The patient may be maintained on lorazepam administered every 4 to 8 hours or, better, switched to a long-acting anticonvulsant. Be prepared to resuscitate the patient.

Side Effects of Lorazepam

Side effects of lorazepam are usually related to its rate of administration and abnormal sensitivity of some patients to the drug. Respiratory depression and decreased level of consciousness can occur. The drug acts synergistically with barbiturates and other sedatives in bringing about these side effects.

Diazepam (Valium)

This benzodiazepine is no more effective in stopping seizures than lorazepam. Its half-life as an antiepileptic medicine is much shorter than as a sedative. A patient may require frequently repeated (every 20–30 min) doses leading to an unacceptable degree of sedation without achieving long-lasting seizure control.

Phenytoin

If the patient has temporarily stopped seizing, phenytoin (Dilantin) is an excellent drug choice. Phenytoin is a relatively safe, long-acting antiepileptic medicine. It may be used alone or in conjunction with lorazepam in the treatment of status epilepticus. It must be given intravenously. The dose is 18 to 20 mg/kg (8–9 mg/lb). Phenytoin is not absorbed after intramuscular administration, and causes muscle necrosis. The advantages of phenytoin include minimal alteration of the level of consciousness, absence of respiratory depression, and a long half-life so that repeated doses are not required for several hours.

Before starting i.v. phenytoin for seizures, it is best to review an EKG (or at least a rhythm strip) to be certain that a significant degree of heart block, bradycardia, acute myocardial infarction, or congestive heart failure does not exist. These are relative, but not absolute, contraindications to the use of the drug. Stopping status epilepticus is even more important in the cardiac-compromised patient. If any cardiac problems do exist, the rate of infusion should be slow; 25 mg/min or less is generally recommended. Death can occur from too rapid an infusion of phenytoin. In most cases (children or adult), administer 18 to 20 mg/kg intravenously at a rate of 50 mg/min (1 ml/min) of the commercially available preparation. Continuous cardiac monitoring and frequent blood pressure checks should be performed, with the physician in immediate attendance. If the blood pressure should drop or arrhythmia develop, the infusion should be stopped and not resumed until cardiac activity has stabilized.

Side Effects of Phenytoin

The side effects of phenytoin are related primarily to the rate of administration of the drug. These include hypotension and cardiac arrhythmia. Blood pressure and EKG should be monitored during infusion. Phenytoin must be used cautiously in the presence of severe arteriosclerotic heart disease, congestive heart failure, second and third degree arteriovenous block, significant bradycardia, advanced age, or history of idiosyncratic reaction.

Calculating Phenytoin Dose (Weight in Kilograms)

Determine patient's weight in kilograms (2.2 lb = 1 kg) and multiply by 18 mg/kg.

Example:

120 lb patient

$$120 \text{ lb} \times \frac{1 \text{ kg}}{2.2 \text{ lb}} = 55 \text{ kg}$$

55 kg x 18 mg/kg = 990 mg

990 mg x 1 ml = 20 ml of a 50 g/ml commercially available phenytoin solution (50 mg for a 120 lb patient)

Administer intravenously at 50 mg/min, injecting at the rate of 1 ml/min.

Calculating Phenytoin Dose (Weight in Pounds)

Determine patient's weight in pounds and multiply by 8 mg/lb.

Example:

120 lb patient
120 lb x 8 mg/lb = 960 mg
960 mg x 1 ml = 19.8 ml of a 50 g/ml commercially available phenytoin solution (50 mg for a 120 lb patient)

Administer intravenously at 50 mg/min, injecting at the rate of 1 ml/min.

Injection of Phenytoin

Phenytoin may be injected undiluted directly into the vein or, alternatively, it may be diluted with half-normal or normal saline (100–200 ml for total dose) and given as an infusion.

1. Start an i.v. line with a volume control set
2. Add 5 ml of 0.45% or 0.9% sodium chloride solution to the set
3. Add the ordered amount of phenytoin injection to the set
4. Add a sufficient volume of 0.45% or 0.9% sodium chloride solution to produce a dilution of 20 to 30 mg of drug/ml of fluid
5. Because minor crystallization has sometimes been noted, it is desirable to place a filter (0.22 or 0.45 microns) on the line
6. Use of an i.v. infusion pump is recommended to ensure an accurate and safe infusion rate

At the time of this writing, a phenytoin prodrug is under active clinical investigation but is not yet approved by the Food and Drug Administration. If this drug comes on the market it will provide a useful way of administering phenytoin parenterally. Unlike Dilantin, the prodrug can be given i.m. for maintenance when patients cannot take oral medicines or are postoperative. It has usefulness in status epilepticus because it can be given intramuscularly or intravenously without concern for the cardiac effects associated with the highly alkaline solution used for phenytoin itself.

Other Drugs

If status epilepticus does not respond to lorazepam or phenytoin administration, it is often an indication of an acute intracerebral lesion or an undiagnosed metabolic cause. Before starting treatment with additional agents, re-evaluate the diagnosis because the cause of the status epilepticus may be as life-threatening as the seizures.

The choice of drug treatment after lorazepam or phenytoin failure is controversial. Some prefer phenobarbital loading (9 mg/kg i.v.) at a rate of 50 mg/min, followed by an additional 9 mg/kg if not effective. This regimen should be used with considerable caution in patients of advanced age, with compromised respiratory function, or with significant metabolic disturbances. This is especially important if diazepam or lorazepam has been used initially because of the risk of cardiorespiratory collapse. Be prepared to intubate the patient at a moment's notice when administering phenobarbital.

Paraldehyde may also be used, but also is no longer readily available. Barbiturate-induced coma, with the dose adjusted to cause a "burst suppression" pattern on the electroencephalogram (EEG), can be used for status epilepticus persisting for more than 6 hr.

CHILDREN AND STATUS EPILEPTICUS

Types of Status Epilepticus in Children

Children, like adults, can have continuous or repetitive generalized tonic-clonic seizures, absence seizures, and simple or complex partial seizures. The relative medical significance is also the same in both children and adults: Generalized tonic-clonic status epilepticus is life-threatening, whereas absence seizures and partial seizures are usually not.

Guidelines for Treatment of Status Epilepticus in Children

1. Preserve respiratory function
2. Diagnose the condition and its cause
3. Promptly obtain specimens for laboratory tests. These should include a blood cell count and baseline values for blood levels of electrolytes, glucose, calcium, blood urea nitrogen, creatinine, and transaminase
4. Consider a lumbar puncture in any febrile child, especially under 18 months of age. Meningitis may occur without "neck stiffness"
5. Measure antiepileptic medicine levels in patients with known seizures
6. Establish an i.v. line
7. Use loading doses of antiepileptic medicines initially (see below)
8. In cases of status epilepticus caused by antiepileptic medicine withdrawal, the treatment of choice is reinstitution of the same drug. This can be done parenterally with phenobarbital and phenytoin. Other major antiepileptic medicines are not available for parenteral use, and may have to be introduced orally

9. Avoid short-acting barbiturates (pentothal and amobarbital), which have no therapeutic advantage and are likely to lead to respiratory arrest
10. There is no single best treatment for status epilepticus in children. Three acceptable choices in wide use are phenytoin, lorazepam, and paraldehyde

DRUG THERAPY FOR STATUS EPILEPTICUS IN CHILDREN

Phenytoin

Administer phenytoin (Dilantin) by the i.v. route only. Intramuscular administration is useless. It causes tissue irritation and the drug is not absorbed into the circulation. The dose in children is 18 to 20 mg/kg (8–9 mg/lb), slowly administered at a rate not exceeding 50 mg/min. Administer as follows:

1. Start an intravenous line with a volume control set
2. Add 5 ml of 0.45% or 0.9% sodium chloride solution to the set
3. Add the required amount of phenytoin injection to the set
4. Add a sufficient volume of 0.45% or 0.9% sodium chloride solution to produce a dilution of 20 to 30 mg of drug/ml of fluid
5. Because minor crystallization has sometimes been noted, it is desirable to place a filter (0.22 to 0.45 microns) on the line
6. Use of an i.v. infusion pump is recommended to ensure an accurate and safe infusion rate

The advantages of phenytoin include minimal alteration in level of consciousness, no respiratory depression, and the establishment of a maintenance dose initially.

Side Effects of Phenytoin

The side effects seen in older patients, including hypotension and cardiac arrhythmia, are rare in children.

Lorazepam

Administer lorazepam (Ativan) intravenously and slowly (intramuscularly is a less desirable choice in children with small muscle mass). For infants and children the dose is 0.05 to 0.1 mg/kg with a maximum dose of 0.2 mg/kg. The patient should be switched to phenytoin or another suitable antiepileptic medicine as soon as convenient. Advantages of lorazepam include:

1. Prolonged antiepileptic activity
2. Rapid onset of action

Side Effects of Lorazepam

Side effects of lorazepam in children include frequent complications of apnea, bradycardia, and hypotension. Cardiac arrest and thrombophlebitis have also been reported. Respiratory embarrassment is more likely to occur in patients who are also receiving barbiturates.

Paraldehyde

Paraldehyde given rectally is both safe and effective. Doses of 0.3 ml/kg are mixed with an equal amount of mineral oil. The dose can be repeated in 20 to 30 min if needed. Paraldehyde is easily administered and ordinarily is safe.

Side Effects of Paraldehyde

Beware of the possibility of using outdated paraldehyde from stock bottles (ampules are a preferred way of storage). Paraldehyde absorption may be unpredictable, particularly if the rectum is filled with stool.

Long-Term Management Of Epilepsy

9

GENERAL PRINCIPLES OF LONG-TERM MANAGEMENT

It is instructive to think of epilepsy as an example of a chronic disease. By definition, a chronic disease is a condition for which there is no quick cure. That means the patient must accept the fact that the aim of treatment is to live successfully with the problem, that it is not going to "go away," and that compromises will have to be made.

In treating chronic disease it is important that we keep the following clearly in mind:

- The need for clear therapeutic aims
- The need for a careful treatment plan
- The need for the patient's cooperation and understanding
- The need for setting decision points in advance

Perhaps the trickiest task is to get the patient to accept that this is indeed a long-term process. That means that the patient must abandon the idea that he can be a passive recipient of treatment and walk out cured in a brief time. Once the patient understands this, it is possible to begin the steps that are necessary for successful treatment.

In treating epilepsy, our aim is no seizures, no side effects, and a healthy outlook on life. It is important to try to get the patient completely seizure free. Patients may be impaired by seizures for only a few minutes a year, but can be totally disabled. The patient with even one or two seizures a year is unable to drive, finds it much harder to obtain employment and educational opportunities, will be discriminated against for both health and life insurance, and will live with constant fear and anxiety.

Therapeutic Aims

The therapeutic aims in the long-term management of a patient with epilepsy are:

- To bring seizures to a complete halt, without toxicity
- To avoid disability, and return the patient to full participation in life
- To avoid anxiety and develop a positive outlook with a sense of being able to cope

To achieve these aims, it is necessary for the physician to spend a substantial amount of time talking with the patient. The patient must understand:

- What is wrong (that he has seizures)
- Why it is wrong (the cause of the seizures)

- What the possibilities are for complete seizure control
- What the prognosis is for a normal life

Establishing a Treatment Plan

The treatment plan must include:

- Coming to an accurate diagnosis and sharing this with the patient
- Choosing an appropriate antiepileptic drug or drugs
- Taking necessary steps to assure the patient's cooperation and understanding

This latter requires no high-tech facility, but does require time and thought. First, patients must be taught the general facts about epilepsy. They want to know about the types of epilepsy, the general types of causes, what tests and treatments are carried out, and about antiepileptic drugs, their use, side effects, and costs.

Using this as a base, teach the patient the specific facts about his problem. He wants to know about the type of epilepsy, the etiology (if known), and the results of the diagnostic tests; what drug is being prescribed, why it is being prescribed, when blood level tests are indicated, and the pharmacokinetics of his specific drug regimen.

We should also teach the patient about keeping a calendar of when seizures occur and when medicines are taken. This permits reconstruction of events to see if, indeed, a failure of compliance is playing a role or if the patient is simply not responding to what we thought was an appropriate antiepileptic drug. A general discussion of nonspecific precipitating factors, such as menstruation, loss of sleep, too much caffeine, stress, etc., and how they raise and lower the seizure threshold is important. The patient wants a prognosis for complete seizure control, whether there are risks of injury or death, and the chances of remission.

Finally, but hardly least, be sure that the patient and the family understand about the first aid for the specific seizures that the patient has and how to recognize and what to do in the case of status epilepticus.

After all this is done, repeat it and then repeat it again on subsequent visits. This information is absolutely necessary if the patient is to participate appropriately in his care, and none of us learns everything the first time.

Once the patient understands the basic facts about his condition, we can help the patient take charge of his life. We can teach better coping skills and provide support during times of situational stress. The patient will become receptive to teaching about compliance, especially when the use of a calendar can show a direct relationship between lack of compliance and the occurrence of seizures.

With the initial choice of antiepileptic drugs, and again subsequently with each change, review with the patient your medication prescription, the half-life of the particular drugs, the dosing interval you are using and why, and what to do in the case of missed doses.

Patients tend to be noncompliant. Those who are doing very well tend to forget their medicines and need to be reminded. Those who are doing poorly think the medicines are useless and don't take the regimen seriously. Both kinds of patients are best handled by random checks of blood levels. Variations of more than ±20% suggest noncompliance and the need for renewed patient education.

One of the most valuable tools that we use at MINCEP Epilepsy Care is a compliance clinic run by a nurse clinician. Patients can come in as frequently as weekly, load their pill boxes under the supervision of the nurse clinician, ask questions, receive reassurance, and learn to participate in a social ritual that encourages long-term compliance with the treatment regimen.

Let the patient help design the dosage regimen for his convenience. Many patients find taking a midday dose difficult. Use b.i.d. (breakfast and dinner or "every time you brush your teeth") dosage wherever possible. It is simple to remember and avoids losing an entire day's dose if pills are taken only once a day.

Pillboxes with seven compartments are helpful. Use two, one for a.m., one for p.m. The patient can tell at a glance whether he remembered to take his medications, and can take a catch-up dose sooner, resulting in less risk of seizures or toxicity.

Addressing Common Concerns

Address common concerns and misunderstandings even if the patient does not voluntarily voice them. Many people have questions that they do not ask, such as:

- If I have seizures does it mean that I am going to go crazy?
- What about taking all these drugs? Am I going to get hooked on them?
- Will I die from a seizure?
- If I have children, will they get epilepsy?
- What about feelings of embarrassment after a seizure?
- Did I get epilepsy from my parents?

It is important to help the patient overcome his sense of helplessness. It is also important that the patient newly diagnosed with seizures be returned to employment as quickly as possible. After 4 to 6 months of unemployment, the likelihood of the patient becoming chronically unemployed or permanently disabled increases substantially.

Education and Recreation

Avoid severe and unnecessary restrictions for the patient. Grade the risks depending on the degree of seizure control and the degree of common sense that the patient displays (see Chapter 4).

A patient is more likely to die from drowning in a bathtub than from an accident at work. Most patients with seizures require few or no limitations.

THE PHYSICIAN'S ROLE

Eliminating Social Stigma

For many years, physicians talked about the so-called epileptic personality. Abnormal behavior may result from the same disturbance in brain function that produces seizures, but the personality problems of the patient with seizures usually result from a downward social spiral. Patients with seizures develop fears and anxiety, which can lead them to withdraw socially. Social withdrawal leads to social isolation, which in turn leads to frustration, anger, and alienation. A frustrated, angry patient is a difficult patient. Often, these factors also lead to personality disorders, neuroses, and psychoses.

It is important not to speak of the patient with seizures as "an epileptic." This tends to make the fact that the patient has seizures more central to individual identity than gender or name. Many patients with intractable seizures have become so isolated from society that they truly think of themselves as "epileptics." Although it takes more words, it is much better to speak of someone who "has epilepsy" or has "recurrent seizures." When the cause of the seizures has been identified, it is better to speak of a patient with a brain scar causing recurrent seizures.

Manipulating Medications and Beyond

Many physicians soon realize that drug management alone does not ensure that patients with epilepsy will be able to learn, work, and live normally. Some children with seizures have physical and cognitive problems requiring coordinated interdisciplinary care. Many youths and young adults face difficult life decisions that are further complicated by their epilepsy. If the physician limits his role to manipulating medications, he falls short of ensuring the patient's well-being.

The physician cannot, and should not, feel responsible for directing all aspects of life for the individual with epilepsy. But the physician *should* take a leadership role within the broader human services system. The experience of MINCEP Epilepsy Care indicates that a large part of disability suffered by most patients with seizures lies in the area of self-esteem and coping. If patients believe that they are of little worth, and if they have no mechanisms with which to cope, they will almost certainly become passive and aimless. Early intervention is necessary to avoid the development of this defeatist attitude. The use of counselors, psychologists, social workers, and group therapy to deal with the problem once it has developed is essential if these patients are to be helped. Patients with seizures are physically impaired only a few minutes to a few hours each year when the seizures are actually occurring, but a great many are totally disabled because of the related social and psychological problems.

Consulting

Schools, vocational agencies, public health programs, and other community agencies often call on the physician for consultation. Providing medical information about epilepsy may help more than in any other way to eliminate unnecessary concerns and restrictions imposed by authorities who may not fully understand seizure disorders.

Referring

Individuals and families rely on the physician's recommendation and endorsement of problems and services. The issues may range from eligibility to attend summer camp to fitness for an occupation. In these cases the physician's knowledge of which specialized programs are available can make an important difference.

Advocacy

It is difficult to change programs, residential opportunities, and vocational plans. The physician's position of leadership in the community gives him a special opportunity to bring about favorable change. Accurate medical knowledge and support is needed if community officials are to be helped to increase options available to individuals with epilepsy.

Addressing Problems Associated with Seizures

In addition to controlling seizures, the physician may need to address certain other problem areas:

- Personal feelings of the patient about seizures, especially poor self-image and social withdrawal
- How the patient deals with these feelings
- How the patient copes with the real problems created by his seizures
- Feelings of the family about seizures
- How family members deal with their feelings and with those of the patient
- Changes in life-style, such as revised safety precautions at home and at work, failure to receive a driver's license, or failure to have a driver's license renewed
- Payment for necessary medical care and medications
- Discrimination in employment

See Chapter 17 for information on where to turn for help.

STOPPING ANTIEPILEPTIC MEDICATIONS IN CHILDREN AND ADULTS WITH EPILEPSY

Many children with epilepsy will be able to go without antiepileptic drugs for the rest of their lives. The problem is to determine which children this applies to and when to cautiously try to wean them from these medicines. As a rule of thumb, the patient should be seizure free for at least 2 years before attempting to stop the antiepileptic drugs. Those patients without neurological signs and without focal abnormalities are most likely to be successfully weaned. Children whose seizures have a clear-cut cause have a higher risk of recurrence than children with idiopathic epilepsy. However, those with a clear-cut cause usually have a higher incidence of other risk factors, such as a long duration of epilepsy, multiple seizure types, and an abnormal electroencephalogram (EEG).

In general, patients who are going to have seizures when medicines are withdrawn are more likely to do so within 6 months to 1 year after the medicines are stopped. Late recurrences do occur, but they are rare and are under 20%.

Similar considerations exist for stopping medicines in adults. Withdrawal of antiepileptic medicine is associated with anywhere from a 10% to 63% risk of seizure relapse. An abnormal EEG, frequent seizures before seizure control, focal neurological deficit, other evidence of brain damage such as mental retardation, and clear-cut symptomatic etiology increase the risk of relapse.

The considerations in stopping antiepileptic drugs in adults are different than in children. In a child under 16 years of age, the recurrence of a seizure is unfortunate but does not necessarily place the child at major social risk. However, an unexpected seizure in an adult who had been seizure free for many years creates many problems with respect to employment, driving, insurability, and self-confidence. Under those circumstances, patients frequently elect to continue on antiepileptic drugs long term if their dose is small and they do not have substantial side effects.

SELECTED READINGS

1. Gumnit RJ. *Living well with epilepsy*. New York: Demos Press, 1990.

2. Gumnit RJ. *Help your child live well with epilepsy*. New York: Demos Press, 1994
3. Shinnar S, Vining EPG, Mellits ED, et al. Discontinuing antiepileptic medication in children with epilepsy after two years without seizures: a prospective study. *N Engl J Med* 1985;313:976–980.

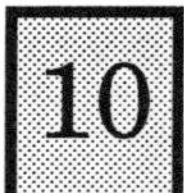

The Difficult Patient
When Seizures Don't Stop

RE-EVALUATING THE DIFFICULT PATIENT

Most patients with uncomplicated seizures can be brought under complete control and will have no further seizures within 90 days from the start of treatment. Using the principle of starting with one drug and increasing the dose to just short of toxicity solves the seizure problem for the great majority of patients. This assumes, of course, that the type of seizure has been properly identified and the appropriate drug has been selected. The difficult patient, therefore, is one who continues to have seizures despite standard treatment.

If the patient continues to have seizures, one of three situations must apply. Either the diagnosis is wrong, the treatment is wrong, or the treatment is theoretically correct but the patient is not complying. This seemingly simple statement provides a clear guide to the orderly thinking that is necessary to come to grips with the patient who is not doing well. The physician faced with a patient who continues to have seizures needs to re-evaluate the diagnosis, the treatment, and patient compliance. At the same time, the physician should do some self-examination. Is she the right physician for this patient at this time? Do they have a good relationship, does the patient trust her, does the patient require the attention of a specialist?

Reviewing the Diagnosis

Is the diagnosis correct? Does the patient have epilepsy or something else? The differential diagnosis with epilepsy includes both physiological and psychological nonepileptic events (see Chapter 11), migraine headaches, breath-holding attacks, etc. The diagnosis of epilepsy can rarely be made with certainty in the absence of capturing one of the seizures with combined video and electroencephalogram (EEG) recording. Nonetheless, most patients can be treated on the basis of a presumptive diagnosis, and if they respond to treatment this is good enough. However, when the seizures don't stop, we must re-examine our diagnosis and go back to fundamentals.

Reviewing Classification

If the patient does indeed have epilepsy, does she have one or more than one kind of seizure? Perhaps the antiepileptic drug chosen is working for one kind of seizure but does not control a second type. Often the patient and the family are unable to make a distinction until the physician has witnessed all the types of seizures on video EEG and can help them make that distinction.

Reviewing Treatment

Is the treatment correct? Table 3.1 provides my approach to selecting antiepileptic drugs approved by the United States Food and Drug Administration for different types of seizures. Refer to this table if you are certain of the diagnosis and the patient is not responding to adequate levels of your chosen antiepileptic drug. Remember, do not treat the blood level, but treat the patient. You cannot be sure that the patient has been tried on adequate dosages of the drug until that drug has been pushed to toxicity.

Do not assume that the drug is ineffective until you have reconsidered the pharmacokinetics of that drug in the context of this particular patient. If the dosing intervals are too long, the drug may be effective for only a portion of the day. Remember that half-lives decrease with polypharmacy and may be decreased by self-induction of certain drugs such as carbamazepine. Try checking both fasting levels and the level just before a subsequent dose. It may answer this question.

Keep in mind that phenytoin (Dilantin) and carbamazepine (Tegretol) occasionally can paradoxically produce seizures if the serum level is too high. The increased levels may occur without signs of clinical toxicity. This problem should be considered if the phenytoin level is over 40 g/ml or the carbamazepine level exceeds 10 g/ml.

Antiepileptic drugs may not be the appropriate treatment. It may be necessary for the patient to undergo surgery for epilepsy. This is best determined by an experienced group of epileptologists at a comprehensive epilepsy center.

Reviewing Compliance

If the patient is not complying with treatment, consider whether or not the patient:

- Understands the need for compliance
- Understands what is necessary to do to achieve compliance

- Wants to comply
- Is permitted to comply

Noncompliance

If the diagnosis is right and the choice of anticonvulsant is right, ask yourself if the patient is compliant. If the patient is not compliant, it is necessary to undertake a different series of maneuvers.

In general, a simple way to determine if the patient is taking the medicine is to measure serum drug levels on three different occasions. Preferably, the blood samples should be taken at the same time of day, and the patient should not be aware that you suspect noncompliance. If the three serum drug levels, measured at the same time in relation to the dose, show variation of greater than 20% among them, the question of poor compliance should be raised.

The patient who does not understand the need for compliance may not have understood the initial explanation. Most people need to hear instructions several times. Or, the patient may have understood exactly what you wanted, but did not understand why it is so important. Such a patient needs to be re-educated. Explain again to the patient what needs to be done and why. It may be worthwhile to have the patient visit your office nurse on several occasions for reinforcement. One helpful maneuver is to have the patient keep a log of the drug she takes, the time she takes it, and when the seizures occur. This reinforces the importance of taking medicines regularly, and helps the patient to draw her own conclusions (see sample form in the Appendix).

The patient may not be able to comply because of psychological incapacity:

Denial. Many patients use denial. They become so anxious over the thought of having seizures and of having to take medicines indefinitely that psychologically the problem becomes too difficult to face. The patient should be confronted, but in a nonthreatening manner. It requires a gradual and gentle approach. The physician is an authority figure and a support structure; to bark suddenly at the patient may be too threatening. On the other hand, it is important to help the patient face reality.

Anger. The patient may become so frustrated and unhappy over the thought of having to take medicines and over the implications of having seizures that she becomes angry. The same phenomenon is seen in patients with juvenile diabetes. If the physician can avoid getting angry in return, the problem usually can be worked out.

Secondary gain. Much more troublesome are the patients who have a substantial amount of secondary gain as a result of having seizures. They get a great deal of attention and their dependency needs are met. For example, perhaps the only way to get financial help from parents or the welfare system is to be disabled. It is necessary to remove the reward and give the patient some other type of gratification. This is easier said than done, especially with the patient whose dependency needs are seemingly limitless.

Often the patient *cannot comply.* She may be of very low intelligence or have severe neurotic or psychotic thinking. Particularly troublesome is the patient with a short memory span. The impaired memory may be the result of the organic brain damage that initially led to seizures, it can be an effect of brain damage and senility in older age, or it may be related to toxic effects of the prescribed antiepileptic medicines. These handicapped patients are usually dependent on other people: parents, spouse, or counselors. It may be necessary to train these other people to help the patient. Simple overlearning techniques to help train the patient are often effective. A week's supply of pills may be laid out in an egg carton or a pillbox. The patient is instructed not to go to bed at night without taking all the pills that are left from that day's section.

If the patient is alcoholic or drug dependent, seizure control can rarely be successfully approached. Rapid changes in metabolism and erratic behavior are to be expected.

Social intervention, and possibly sheltered living, may be necessary before seizures can be brought under control.

There are patients who live in such deprived conditions that they cannot afford to buy their anticonvulsant medication. Others find that their antiepileptic medicines are frequently stolen to be sold on the street. The physician should turn to social agencies for help with these problems.

Managing Noncompliance

The physician can manage noncompliance in several ways:

1. When the patient is uninformed:

   Use patient education materials
   Use staff members as a resource for patient education
   Check to see if the patient actually understood the explanation given at the previous visit

2. When the patient is psychologically noncompliant:

   Remove rewards for inappropriate behavior seeking secondary gain
   Give rewards for appropriate behavior

3. When the patient uses denial:

   Confront the patient in a nonthreatening manner
   Use a gradual and gentle approach
   Provide emotional support but also provide reality

4. When the patient cannot comply:

   Identify the problem and work with those who care for the patient so that they may be able to help her comply

5. If the patient is alcoholic or drug dependent:

   Seizure control cannot be approached while the patient is drug dependent and metabolism is fluctuating rapidly
   Consider recommending social intervention or sheltered living

One of the most effective techniques for helping a patient take her medicine regularly is close attention. Experience at MINCEP Epilepsy Care shows that if patients are seen frequently, as often as once a week, by a nurse, compliance rapidly improves. The nurses emphasize the importance of taking the medicine regularly. They help the patients count their pills for each day and, if necessary, help the patients put them into a pillbox or egg carton. The patient can readily check before going to bed if they took the day's dosage. Patients appear to respond to having someone care. It may not be practical for the physician to see the patient this often, but someone in the physician's office can. The cost of these regular visits is small compared to the cost of hospitalization when seizures go out of control.

DETAILED STRATEGY FOR MANAGING
NONCOMPLIANCE

Whether or not a patient complies is the result of many different forces. Behavior modification techniques must be developed individually for each patient. Regardless of the techniques employed, increased individual attention by nurse, physician, or other health professional seems to be crucial. Although there are several strategies and techniques that can be employed, all depend on monitoring by the treating team so that the patient is given objective facts about her behavior. The patient loses trust in the physician if she is accused of noncompliance because drug metabolism has been changed by the introduction of other medications or if the laboratory fails to provide accurate measurement of drug levels.

The most common behavioral modification techniques are reminders of proper behavior. This can be done verbally. Instructions are given on each visit about taking the medicines and when to take them. More helpful is the use of calendars, individualized medication programs, and pillboxes.

Progressively Shaping Behavior

The patient must understand at the outset that the behavior eventually expected is complete self-medication. Many patients, especially those of limited intelligence, have to be helped to develop appropriate responses through a series of successive steps. For example, help them pack their pillboxes on weekly visits to the office. Then, have them do it at home and bring them in to show how well they have done. Eventually, they can do it on their own. Each step must be reinforced, and no further steps taken until the previous one is mastered.

Health Education

First, patients with seizures have to learn what acceptable health behavior is. The more the patients understand their illness, the more initiative they can take. Thus, they can begin to take an active role in tailoring dosage intervals to suit their own individual life-style and make changes in their activities to maximize seizure control.

Reinforcement

The basic principles of behavior modification apply to obtaining compliance. In general, try to use only positive reinforcement. Minimizing approach-avoidance conflict makes the patient's visit to the physician or nurse a positive experience. Reinforcement must be given as soon as good behavior is observed, in small and frequent amounts. Encourage positive reinforcement from the family and peers as well.

General Stressors

There may be stresses that lower the seizure threshold, including:

- Anxiety
- Water-loading
- Lack of sleep or excessive fatigue
- Poor diet
- Blood sugar variations
- Interactions with other prescribed drugs such as antihistamines or aminophylline
- Interactions with other nonprescribed drugs such as caffeine, "angel dust," strychnine, amphetamines, PCB, and other street drugs sold as "speed" or "uppers"

Referral to a Neurologist

If the patient continues to have seizures after 3 months of adequate blood levels of a major antiepileptic medicine, she probably has unique, highly specialized needs. It is best to get help early to avoid disability. Certainly, if the seizures persist after 6 months, the family physician should refer the patient to a neurologist. If the patient has uncontrolled seizures for 6 months or more, and especially if she is forced out of work, it becomes extremely difficult to get her back into the mainstream of society.

Refer the difficult patient to a neurologist under the following circumstances:

- Uncertainty about the diagnosis. Are the episodes true seizures, cardiac difficulty, or some other problem?
- Uncertainty about the cause of seizures. If the problem is definitely a seizure, is it caused by a brain tumor, infection, or something else that needs immediate treatment?
- The existence of focal neurological signs. These imply focal brain damage and increase anxiety about the underlying cause.
- Failure to achieve complete seizure control within 3 months. Lack of seizure control raises the question about mistakes in diagnosis or treatment, or the patient may have severe epilepsy that needs specialized care.

- Change in the type of seizure. A change in the seizure pattern raises the question of an active brain process, which requires evaluation. Other factors, such as changes in the body's metabolism of drugs, also may have to be evaluated.
- An increase in seizure frequency with an unchanged antiepileptic medicine level. This suggests an active process, which should be carefully evaluated.
- Increase in physical or emotional disability of the patient. Referral is warranted to prevent further deterioration.

If the patient is still having seizures after you have re-evaluated the situation, consider an early referral to a specialized epilepsy center. Early intervention is best. The sooner the patient is adequately treated, the less disability she will have. But, in addition, it is my belief that the longer patients have seizures, the more likely they are to become particularly difficult to treat. Also, for all practical purposes, surgery will not be appropriately evaluated without a referral to a specialized epilepsy center. For some reason, in our health care system in the United States today, patients are not being referred for surgery in a timely fashion. The average patient undergoing surgery at MINCEP Epilepsy Care has had seizures for 14 years. We don't allow people to have gall bladder attacks for 14 years, so why do we let them have seizures for 14 years?

SELECTED READINGS

1. Gumnit RJ, Leppik IE. The epilepsies. In: Rosenberg RN, ed. *Comprehensive neurology*. New York: Raven Press, 1991: 311–336.
2. Leppik IE. Variability of antiepileptic medication concentration and compliance. In: Cramer, JA, Spilker B, eds. *Patient compliance in medical practice and clinical trials*. New York: Raven Press, 1991.
3. Schmidt D, Leppik IE. Compliance in epilepsy. *Epilepsy Research*. Amsterdam: Elsevier, 1988 (suppl 1).

11   Nonepileptic Events

Over the years, a broad range of conditions have been lumped together under a variety of names: hysterical seizures, pseudoseizures, nonepileptic seizures, nonepileptic events, and psychogenic seizures. Patients with this problem are difficult to diagnose and treat, but they are not uncommon. They represent 20% of the referrals to a specialized epilepsy center like MINCEP Epilepsy Care. Because they are frequently diagnosed and treated inadequately, they use an inappropriate amount of medical resources, not only in the form of visits to physicians' offices, but also to emergency rooms and by hospitalization.

Nonepileptic events that at first appear to be seizures can be divided into physiological events, psychogenic events, malingering, and misdiagnosis (Fig. 11.1).

Numerous studies have proved that there is no single presentation of nonepileptic events. The diagnosis cannot be made with certainty on the basis of any one characteristic, or even on the basis of a single electroencephalogram (EEG) recorded during the ictus.

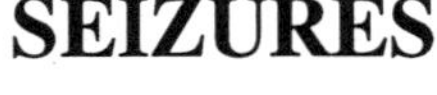

SEIZURES

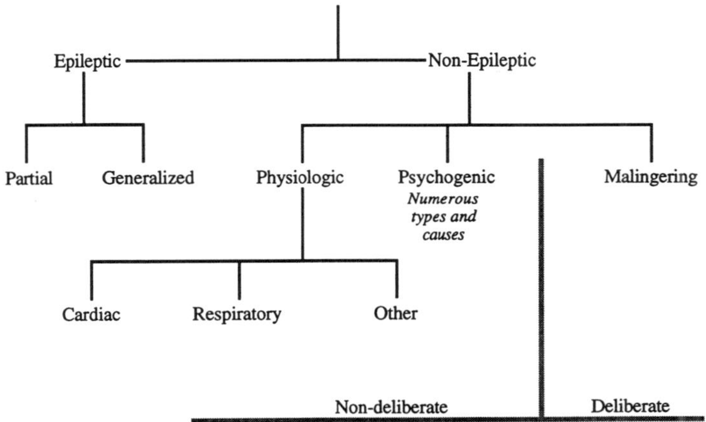

Deliberate: With intent to deceive or consciously influence observer.

Figure 11.1.

PHYSIOLOGICAL NONEPILEPTIC EVENTS

Psychogenic seizures rarely begin in children under the age of 6 years, and rarely start in middle or old age. Many cardiac and respiratory causes of physiological nonepileptic events occur later in life.

Disturbances of consciousness produced by decreased oxygen tension to the brain may be produced by the following conditions and cause behavior that mimics psychogenic or true seizures:

1. Problems in perfusion: rhythm disturbance (e.g., Stokes-Adams disease), transient ischemic attacks, emboli from carotid plaques
2. Decreased oxygen tension from poor saturation: pneumonia, coma, lung shunts, pulmonary emboli
3. Metabolic causes: decreased blood glucose levels, electrolyte shifts

4. Toxicity: street drugs or prescription drugs, alcohol intoxication. A particularly troubling event may be toxic reaction to excessive concentrations of antiepileptic drugs from erratic absorption

MALINGERING

Malingerers rarely present at specialized epilepsy centers, but may be a real problem in the primary care setting, especially if the patient is forced to seek treatment by the courts, a spouse, or an employer. Prisoners and those in military service are particularly likely to be malingerers. Malingerers have, on occasion, mimicked generalized tonic-clonic seizures so well that even experienced epileptologists have been confused. Video/EEG recordings of the events, at least during the ictus, are mandatory for the diagnosis. The absence of postictal slowing during the recovery phase is often helpful.

MISDIAGNOSIS

Misdiagnosis by a physician, nurse, parent, or other caregiver is the most common form of confusion. If the patient accepts a misdiagnosis, he will report frequent seizures and the physician will be tempted to use ever-increasing doses of antiepileptic drugs for what may simply be a misinterpretation of a normal physiological sensation or some benign psychological issue. Mentally retarded individuals often exhibit motor mannerisms, and the patient may be described as having many seizures per day.

PSYCHOGENIC NONEPILEPTIC SEIZURES

The diagnosis of a psychogenic nonepileptic seizure can be made only with the help of video/EEG recordings during the ictus. At the same time, testing of consciousness and reaction to startle response should be carried out. The diagnosis cannot be made on a single event; often the first impression may be wrong.

Patients with true epileptic seizures may occasionally experience a psychogenic seizure during video/EEG monitoring out of a desire to be helpful. Unless the witnessed psychogenic seizure is identical to the presenting problem, a false diagnosis will be made.

Secondary gain plays a role in psychogenic seizures under almost any circumstance, but tends to serve as a reinforcer rather than an etiologic agent *per se*. The etiology of psychogenic seizures can be classified as follows:

- Misdiagnosis-misinterpretation by patient, caregiver/ parent, or physician
- Elaboration: A simple sensory or motor seizure is followed by a more obvious and elaborate psychogenic seizure

The usual etiologies for elaboration are fear, attention-seeking, reinforcement of a dependent role, or a conditioned response. By far, most patients use psychogenic seizures as an inappropriate coping strategy. The patient may have limited intellectual resources, serious psychological conflict, or personality or characterologic issues may be at work.

The experience at MINCEP Epilepsy Care and several peer-reviewed reports indicates that physical and sexual abuse can play an etiologic role in psychogenic seizures, especially in female patients. Female patients are three times more likely to have psychogenic seizures than male patients.

One can often provoke a psychogenic seizure by suggesting that the patient will have a seizure. However, simply because a psychogenic seizure occurred, one cannot conclude that this is the event that prompted the patient to seek medical care. The witnessed event must be compared carefully with the presenting complaint. I do not advocate the injection of a placebo to provoke seizures. In my experience it gives too many false positive results.

THE ROLE OF SERUM HORMONE AND ENZYME MEASUREMENTS

Certain serum hormone and enzyme determinations can be used to separate psychogenic seizures from true epilepsy. However, they are useful only in severe, full-blown seizures that appear to be generalized tonic-clonic. From a practical point of view, obtaining the specimen in a timely manner and the interpretation may be difficult.

Because all these hormones have circadian fluctuations, control values must be based on samples drawn from the patient at the same time of day when no event has taken place. The concentrations go up and down so rapidly that the measurement has to be made during the peak.

Serum prolactin levels drawn 5 to 15 min after a generalized tonic-clonic seizure can be compared to one 90 to 120 min later. A rise of 2 1/2 times control provides about 90% reliability in determining a true generalized tonic-clonic seizure. A negative result has no value in distinguishing complex partial seizures (40% false negative rate).

TREATMENT

Treatment of psychogenic seizures is complex and time-consuming. If treatment is to be successful, the diagnosis must be accurate, or the physician must be willing to risk being wrong and act with great confidence. Any ambivalence provides an opportunity for denial or further manipulation by the patient. Delay the diagnosis until you are certain; a premature diagnosis creates a loss of confidence that may never be overcome.

Because nonepileptic seizures have diverse causes, treatment must be tailored individually. Misdiagnosis is fairly easy to treat if the patient has confidence in your new diagnosis. Anxious patients who misinterpret normal sensations may need a comprehensive approach based on reassurance. Misinterpretation by the caregiver is best approached by educating and reassuring the patient. However, if the caregiver has psychological needs that are met by the misdiagnosis, prolonged counseling and family therapy may be necessary.

Psychogenic seizures are learned behavior. Proper treatment centers on the patient's ability to learn new coping skills. The patient with limited intellectual resources often resorts to psychogenic seizures as a way of avoiding conflict or to influence a highly structured and restricted environment. In that case, treatment is directed at the family and the caregiver.

Patients whose psychogenic seizures arise from psychological conflict or personality or character disorders are the most difficult to treat. They require a team of professionals skilled in the techniques of modern psychology and psychiatry. My experience is that ad hoc task forces created from general hospital support staff do not achieve comparable rates of success. Simply informing the patient that the seizures are nonepileptic is not treatment. Denial and doubt are routine, and are often healthy responses that are necessary for patients who require more time to process the diagnosis. Patients whose nonepileptic seizures represent a significant psychological defense mechanism cannot simply be told the diagnosis. Leaving such patients defenseless without providing alternative coping mechanisms can be and has been catastrophic. Suicide attempts occur, and are occasionally successful.

The treatment of psychogenic seizures requires extensive resources, an experienced team, and a lot of time. It is usually better not to tell the patient of your suspicions. Refer the patient to a specialized epilepsy center and let it make the diagnosis and provide the necessary psychological and psychiatric care at the time the diagnosis is made.

SELECTED READING

1. Gumnit RJ. Psychogenic seizures. In: Wyllie E, ed. *The treatment of epilepsy: principles and practice.* Philadelphia: Lea & Febiger, 1992:692–697.

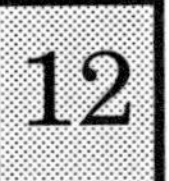 # Specialized Epilepsy Centers

Physicians properly ask why they should refer a patient to a specialized epilepsy center. What can a center do for my patient that I can't do, especially since a specialized epilepsy center sounds expensive? If a patient is completely free of seizures without toxicity and is getting along fine in the community, there is certainly no reason to consider a referral. But even one seizure a year may create major difficulties for a person in terms of employment, driving, insurance, and other important elements of life. A specialized epilepsy center can bring together the combined efforts of a multispecialty team with a great deal of expertise in epilepsy, which has access to specialized equipment that is not generally available in the community. If this is coupled with a genuine desire to heal the patient and not just stop seizures, a great deal of benefit can result.

In fact, I urge early referral. The longer a patient has seizures, the more fixed the disability becomes, and the more difficult it is to turn around her life. In addition, seizures that have been uncontrolled for many years are much harder to bring under control than seizures that are treated vigorously and early. Subtle changes appear to take place in the brain that gradually lower the seizure threshold and, it is thought by some epileptologists, can create secondary epileptic foci elsewhere in the brain.

WHAT TO EXPECT FROM A SPECIALIZED EPILEPSY CENTER

If you refer a patient to a specialized epilepsy center, you should expect that center to provide you and your patient with:

1. An accurate diagnosis of whether or not the patient has epilepsy or some other physiological or psychological problem, or a mixture
2. An accurate diagnosis or classification of the type of seizure or seizures so that an appropriate prognosis and treatment plan can be arrived at
3. A treatment plan that clearly spells out your role in long-term treatment. The patient is best treated by a team of family doctor and epileptologist
4. A thorough evaluation of the psychological and social factors at work in the patient, short-term intervention when appropriate, and assistance in helping the patient get long-term help at home
5. A well thought out treatment program for psychogenic seizures
6. An experienced, comprehensive surgical treatment program
7. A willingness on the part of the epilepsy center to provide long-term consultation and follow-up with you in managing the case. The center help if and when the patient gets into acute difficulties and should provide a ready source of information and support for what is a long-term chronic disease

To do this, the center needs a dedicated multispecialty team of neurologists, psychologists, psychiatrists, clinical neurophysiologists, neuropsychologists, pharmacists, social workers, and nurses. This team should operate a coordinated outpatient/inpatient program and have access to a dedicated inpatient unit for video/EEG recording.

HOW TO CHOOSE A SPECIALIZED
EPILEPSY CENTER

Everything that has the name "specialized epilepsy center" may not be able to deliver the services that are needed. The name on the door may only be advertising. Most physicians search among possible consultants until they find consultants whose opinion they trust, who achieve closure for a clinical problem, and with whom they are comfortable. The same holds true for a specialized epilepsy center. Some of the pitfalls to guard against are those centers that are so excited about epilepsy surgery that they "operate on anything that moves." The hallmark of a good surgeon is knowing when not to operate. At the other end of the spectrum are those centers that are so inexperienced with surgery, or are so afraid of surgery, that they rarely operate. Often many patients that could be helped are told that nothing can be done for them, whereas they could achieve significant help elsewhere. Many small centers springing up around the country lack a sufficient depth of expertise, and tend to handle only easy cases. If they handle the easy cases well and help patients get more advanced help elsewhere, they can do a lot of good. Unfortunately, the natural human tendency is to believe that if you can't help the patient, nobody else can.

There is no nationally recognized certification for epilepsy centers at the time of this writing (Spring, 1994). For information on those centers that have joined the National Association of Epilepsy Centers you can write the National Association of Epilepsy Centers at 5775 Wayzata Blvd., Suite 255, Minneapolis, MN 55416 or telephone 612/525-4526.

SELECTED READING

1. National Association of Epilepsy Centers. Recommended guidelines for diagnosis and treatment in specialized epilepsy centers. *Epilepsia* 1990;31(suppl 1).

<table><tr><td>13</td><td># Surgery For Epilepsy</td></tr></table>

Surgery can be a safe and effective treatment for many patients with epilepsy. It carries risk, it is not foolproof, and it should not be rushed into, nor should it be unduly delayed. But because of recent advances, surgery has become an option physicians are considering more often.

Epilepsy surgery has markedly improved the quality of life for many people who have lived with the ongoing trauma of uncontrolled seizures, suffered toxic side effects from medications, or, for other reasons, reacted unfavorably to anticonvulsants. But surgical treatment should not be entered into lightly.

A patient whose seizures have not been brought under complete control within 1 year should be referred to an experienced comprehensive epilepsy center for diagnosis and a choice among medical and surgical therapies. Early intervention is important. The longer seizures persist uncontrolled, the harder they are to treat. If children go to school, especially if they go through adolescence, with uncontrolled seizures, the more likely they are to have serious psychological and social problems. The longer an adult is disabled, the harder it is to return to the workplace.

Once a comprehensive epilepsy center has determined that the patient has epilepsy, the precise type of seizure, and that appropriate antiepileptic medications have been tried in adequate dosages, that patient may be considered for epilepsy surgery. However, the patient must be physically and psychologically capable of coping with surgery. That capability should be ascertained before further work-up is undertaken. The presurgical work-up is not always a prolonged or expensive process, but serious mistakes happen if any of the steps are overlooked.

In general, patients to be considered for surgery must be medically refractory. A simple working definition of medical intractability is that the patient has been tried on adequate levels (ideally pushed to toxicity) of at least two or three of the major antiepileptic drugs that are appropriate for the type of seizures that are causing disability.

INDICATIONS FOR SURGERY

General Criteria

Surgery is recommended for patients whose seizures are medically refractory. In addition, the seizures must be drop attacks or be stereotypic and arising from a part of the brain that is amenable to surgical treatment.

EVALUATION PROCESS

Initial Evaluation (Extracranial Evaluation)

The initial evaluation process includes several different examinations designed to detect focal electrophysiological, structural, and functional brain pathology. The electrophysiological assessment is accomplished by obtaining a large sample of the patient's interictal electroencephalogram (EEG) and by recording a sample of the patient's typical seizures by means of time-linked video/EEG recordings. This information serves as the cornerstone of the diagnostic process. The electrophysiological assessment is supplemented by a careful search for a focal structural brain lesion using high-resolution magnetic resonance imaging (MRI) technique. Further evidence of focal brain dysfunction may be revealed by thorough neuropsychological testing and by the results of the intracarotid sodium Amytal study. Selected patients may need further assessment of focal brain dysfunction, which can be provided by positron emission tomography (PET scanning).

The initial evaluation thus consists of a search for converging lines of evidence indicating predominant pathology in one brain region, combined with an assessment of the safety of a surgical treatment directed at that brain region. Approximately 75% of potential surgical candidates can be offered the option of a surgical treatment after their initial evaluation. The other 25% of potential surgical candidates will require additional study after their initial evaluation before a decision regarding surgical treatment can be made.

Because patients must be taken off antiepileptic drugs to record seizures, patients must be attended by specially trained nurses in one of its dedicated special care units, where experienced epileptologists are close at hand.

Intracranial Evaluation

A minority of potential surgical candidates will need a period of intracranial electrophysiological evaluation before surgical treatment. There are basically two indications for intracranial study: (a) the need for clearer definition of the source of seizures and/or (b) the need for careful physiological study of brain regions surrounding the area of proposed brain resection in order to map vital areas of the cortex such as speech and motor areas (functional cortical mapping). In every instance, the results of the initial evaluation must be used to formulate specific questions that can then be answered with intracranial recording procedures.

A variety of techniques can be used for intracranial recording purposes. Subdural strips or grids of electrodes may be placed over the surface of the brain. Depth electrodes may be placed into deep or relatively inaccessible locations by means of stereotactic technique. There is no single best approach for all clinical situations. The best approach in an individual case is that approach that can most likely answer the specifically formulated questions and that presents the least risk for the patient.

MINCEP Epilepsy Care has reduced the percentage of patients requiring intracranial recording by half (to about 25%) since 1990 with a decrease in risk and no apparent worsening in outcome.

SPECIFIC SURGICAL PROCEDURES
AND THEIR INDICATIONS

Anterior Temporal Lobectomy

Anterior temporal lobectomy is the most common surgical treatment for refractory epilepsy. Most patients with refractory epilepsy have complex partial seizures, and most complex seizures arise from the temporal lobe. Therefore, temporal lobectomy is the most common surgical procedure for epilepsy.

Best Candidates for Temporal Lobectomy

Ideal candidates (and often the easiest to identify) are patients with stereotypic complex partial seizures and a consistent unilateral anterior temporal spike or sharp wave focus on the interictal EEG. Magnetic resonance imaging evidence of hippocampal atrophy on the same side is helpful. There are patients who do not meet these criteria who can be successfully treated with surgery, and thus failure to meet these ideal criteria should not preclude a referral.

Extratemporal Cortical Resections (Especially Frontal and Parietal)—Topectomies

Some patients have a seizure focus in the frontal or parietal lobes. These patients cannot be helped by temporal lobectomies. Once again, seizure type and localization must be precisely identified. Surgical resection of these foci usually requires a subdural electrode array for functional cortical mapping.

No resection is performed without carefully weighing all relevant evidence, including neuropsychological studies and functional imaging.

Sectioning the Corpus Callosum

Today, sectioning the corpus callosum is performed more and more often. It is especially recommended for patients suffering from drop attacks. Drop attacks, which may be tonic, atonic, or myclonic, are notoriously resistant to treatment with antiepileptic drugs. Although those suffering from tonic drop attacks have the best chance of benefiting from surgery, patients experiencing other types of drop attacks may also be helped with surgery.

The earlier the patients with drop attacks are identified and operated on, the greater the likelihood of success. Patients suffering from drop attacks frequently injure themselves and accumulate brain damage from head injuries. Early intervention can reduce this trauma. Any patient who suffers drop attacks and has been injured during a seizure should be referred for treatment.

Again, precise knowledge of the type(s) of seizures and the EEG correlate is needed before selecting a patient for treatment. A determination about surgery can often be made by recording just a few seizures. Intracranial recording is not necessary.

Although the procedure does not ordinarily bring about complete control of seizures, it can dramatically reduce the number and severity of drop attacks and eliminate the need for toxic doses of multiple antiepileptic drugs.

The earlier patients with drop attacks are identified and operated on, the greater the likelihood of success. Patients frequently injure themselves, and early intervention reduces a lot of pain. All patients who have drop attacks and have injured themselves during a seizure should be considered for referrals. The patient's IQ and ability to live independently are not overriding considerations in selecting patients for surgery. The primary aims are to stop the injury resulting from abrupt drops, and to reduce the toxicity resulting from high doses of multiple antiepileptic drugs. Sectioning the corpus callosum does not usually bring about complete control of seizures. In particular, it is of no use for the complex partial seizures that many of these patients also have.

HEMISPHERECTOMY

A small but significant number of patients, usually children in the 2- to 14-year-old age group, suffer from frequent, uncontrollable, debilitating seizures involving only one side of the body. These patients are hemiparetic or hemiplegic and have little functional use of the fingers of the affected arm. Even when the left hemisphere is involved, speech is rarely affected (having developed on the other side of the brain). The insults causing this problem appear to occur in utero or in very early infancy. Magnetic resonance imaging studies will usually reveal widespread brain damage in one hemisphere and a relatively normal-appearing brain in the other.

Many of these children can be helped to have complete control of seizures with no worsening of motor movement, and often with marked improvement in their ability to learn. The operation of choice is a modified hemispherectomy. Parts of the diseased brain are left intact to prevent wide shifting of the intracranial contents and subsequent development of complications from frequent small post-traumatic bleeds. However, the sick brain is effectively disconnected from the intact brain, greatly reducing the negative influence of the abnormal electrical discharges occurring from the damaged hemisphere. Early intervention is particularly important in these cases.

CLINICAL PEARL HEMISPHERECTOMY

Patients whose seizures involve one side of the brain, who have little functional use of the fingers of the opposite side of the body, and who are disabled by their frequency of seizures as well as the toxicity of antiepileptic drugs, should be referred for surgical consideration. Patients often improve dramatically in their general learning and behavior skills after hemispherectomy. Early intervention is particularly important in these cases.

RASMUSSEN'S SYNDROME

A small number of young children develop what appears to be a focal encephalitis with debilitating seizures and gradual destruction of their mental and physical abilities. These children do not respond to antiepileptic medications. They should be referred early, and surgery should be considered early in the course of the disease to prevent paralysis, dementia, and death. Any child with uncontrolled seizures, especially with the development of focal neurological signs, should be referred for evaluation soon, certainly within 6 months of onset, and a careful watch should be kept for progressive increase in neurological disability.

WEST'S SYNDROME OR INFANTILE SPASMS

Recent reports indicate that some patients with infantile spasms can be helped with surgical intervention. The surgery performed is essentially a cortical resection, or topectomy. Any child with West's syndrome who has not responded to the usual treatment and has a structural lesion on the MRI should be considered for early surgery. Without MRI findings a much more complex analysis of background EEG and the necessity for PET scan exists. Only a few centers in the United States have experience with this kind of surgery.

SUBPIAL RESECTION OR RAKING

Subpial resection is still under investigation. It has been recommended for patients with epilepsy that arises in the speech or motor areas. If you have a patient with these problems you should consult a reputable comprehensive epilepsy program for advice on the current state of the art.

OUTCOMES

Seventy percent of patients with complex partial seizures who can be operated on without invasive recording are rendered seizure free, and altogether more than 90% are improved (in the experience of MINCEP Epilepsy Care). If depth electrodes or subdural arrays (grids) are needed, 50% are seizure free overall, and 75% are helped. Operations on extratemporal structures are statistically somewhat less successful, but the outcomes are good in properly selected individuals.

SELECTED READINGS

1. Gumnit RJ. Selection of adult patients for surgical treatment of epilepsy. *Acta Neurol Scand* 1988;78(S117):42–46.
2. Theodore WH. Surgical treatment of epilepsy. *Epilepsy Research*. Amsterdam: Elsevier, 1992 (suppl 5).

Epilepsy and Health Insurance

There is hardly a more important topic for the patient with epilepsy than how to pay for treatment. For most Americans, health insurance is how we pay for medical care. However, the health insurance scene in the United States in the spring of 1994 is insane. The existing system is full of artificial barriers to care and coverage. Strong political forces are at work to change the system, but the picture is so confused that no one can accurately predict what health insurance and health care will look like even 3 years from now. This chapter attempts to give a primer about health insurance issues in the United States in early 1994. The reader is reminded that this is a snapshot, and that by the time the book is printed changes will have occurred.

In theory, health insurance is sold in an open market. That means that a willing buyer should have choices among several willing sellers of this necessary service if they can agree on a price. In fact, there are major barriers to obtaining any kind of health insurance for many people, especially those with epilepsy. Insurance companies compete on the basis of price and try to minimize their expenses by practicing adverse selection and redlining. That means they will not insure certain segments of the market (e.g., food service workers) and they will discriminate against certain members of an employee group (e.g., those with chronic disease such as epilepsy). By selling at a rock-bottom price to large employee groups, they preclude the possibility of spreading the risk across a large population (the very essence of the concept of insurance) and therefore charge such high premiums to individuals and small groups that health insurance becomes unaffordable.

There are several approaches to buying health insurance or health care in the United States today. Conventional indemnity health insurance is the classic form but it is rapidly disappearing from the market. With an indemnity policy, insurance companies will pay any licensed physician and hospital for services that are medically necessary. Games are played about medical necessity, as well as the amount that the insurance company is willing to reimburse (artificially set "usual and customary fees," arbitrarily imposed fee schedules). Nonetheless, indemnity insurance provides the greatest opportunity to choose among physicians and to obtain highly specialized services. One way to minimize cost is to look for a policy with a high deductible. This forces the individual to self-insure for predictable day-to-day costs, but provides a reasonable premium for big problems. Good insurance is difficult for an individual to buy, so attempt to obtain it through employment wherever possible.

To control costs and compete on the basis of a lower premium (but in all actuality not much lower), various types of prepayment plans have been created. So-called IPOs (independent practice organizations) and PPOs (preferred provider organizations) restrict the patient to using certain physicians who have agreed to take a lesser reimbursement rate. IPOs and PPOs often require prior approval for all kinds of treatment. Health maintenance organizations (HMOs) are supposed to provide all kinds of health care, including preventive care and prescriptions, for a fixed amount each month without deductible or co-pay. More recently, deductibles and co-pays have been introduced into HMOs. HMOs may be of the closed staff model, in which the physicians are all employed and the patient may have relatively little choice, or the open staff model, in which case the HMO contracts with a variety of physicians throughout a community and the patient may have greater choice. A more recent development has been to combine HMO insurance with the opportunity to go out of plan and go to any physician, in which case the patient is asked to pay a hefty portion of the total cost (typically 20–30%, if they go out of plan).

For the patient with epilepsy there are some specific barriers of particular concern. Managed care concepts have now penetrated health care almost universally. If the HMO or insurance company is relatively unsophisticated, the need for expensive comprehensive treatment for patients with intractable epilepsy may not be recognized. It may be necessary for the patient and physician both to become outspoken advocates if the patient is to get proper help. Contracts between managed care organizations and primary care physicians often place the primary care doctor at risk for expenditures considered excessive by the plan. This tends to inhibit the primary care doctor from referring the patient to a specialist or specialized epilepsy program because such care is perceived as being expensive, and will come out of the referring doctor's income. Equally pernicious is the attitude of some physicians that they know what is best for the patient to the point that they become paternalistic. Some physicians refuse to refer patients for treatment that they want. This is particularly a problem in Britain and Canada, but pervasive throughout the United States as well.

In some parts of the United States, overprescribing and providing too many services continue to be problems, although this is rapidly diminishing. Patients should be careful of physicians who seem to order the same tests over and over again without a clear reason to do so, or who order many different kinds of medicines. Overprescribing in the sense of performing surgery on patients who may not need it is becoming a bigger problem, as more centers for epilepsy surgery develop and they become eager to meet their growth and income goals.

Patients who are totally disabled with epilepsy and are covered by Medicare, or those who have no money and are covered by Medical Assistance or Medicaid, have a particularly difficult problem in obtaining adequate care. The fees paid to physicians by these two programs are relatively small; in some states they do not even cover the physicians' overhead expenses. Many physicians with busy practices do discriminate against patients on Medicare and Medicaid. Many of the comprehensive epilepsy programs find that they cannot provide services to patients on Medicare and Medicaid because the payments are so low that they would be forced out of business.

What advice can be given to a patient with epilepsy under these circumstances? Try to get some sophisticated advice from knowledgeable people in your home community who are familiar with what is going on in your town. Hospital social workers are often a good source. Become strong advocates for governmental regulations requiring community rating and no discrimination against patients with pre-existing conditions. Do not passively accept a refusal by a managed care organization to provide you with specialized epilepsy care. Complain, demand, and ask for support from your physician, your local state legislator, and your local congressman. The provision of medical care in the United States has become a political game. It is a political game even though many of the players are businessmen and bureaucrats and not elected officials. Political games are not won by passively accepting "no" for an answer.

Epilepsy and the Law

15

In the United States, law affects the life of everyone in myriad ways. An overlapping series of local ordinances and state and federal law often create apparent contradictions. The law is constantly changing and no brief discussion of the subject, which is all there is space for here, can hope to cover the subject in detail.

People with epilepsy have historically been discriminated against in the United States and find themselves particularly vulnerable to law in a wide variety of areas of normal life. An excellent introduction to this subject, with many important details and references, is the publication "The Legal Rights of Persons with Epilepsy," published by the Epilepsy Foundation of America in 1992 (see reference section of this chapter).

Patients with epilepsy may find themselves involved in issues of family law, including adoption and child custody, particularly about concerns that their condition will interfere with their ability to be a good parent. They may be caught up in the criminal justice system, by being arrested for seizure-related behavior or by being arrested by carrying medicines prescribed for their disorder, and may need to know their rights as inmates in correctional facilities.

The prevalence of epilepsy among prisoners is much higher than that reported for the general population.

Patients with epilepsy frequently encounter difficulties with employment, both in hiring and firing. They need to understand how their disorder impacts on Worker's Compensation insurance and vocational rehabilitation, as well as the impact of the Rehabilitation Act of 1973 and the Americans with Disabilities Act.

Because people with epilepsy are often disabled, they need to know about Social Security disability benefits and Medicare and Medicaid benefits. Epilepsy may impact on a military career and people with epilepsy who have been in the military must be aware of their rights for veteran's benefits.

Patients with epilepsy have special legal rights to access to education, especially at the elementary school level.

Patients with epilepsy may have problems with public accommodations and may have rights to assistance with public housing.

The area of law that affects everyone with epilepsy and is most important for them to understand deals with access to the health care system (Chapter 14) and with driving (Chapter 16).

We have come a long way! The major book discussing epilepsy and the law in 1966 discussed such issues as eugenic marriage laws, eugenic sterilization laws, commitment to state institutions, and epilepsy as grounds for refusal for admission and immigration to the United States.

ACCESS TO HEALTH CARE

A broad outline of this problem is presented in Chapter 14. Anyone with epilepsy or who has a friend or relative with epilepsy would be well served by carefully evaluating the impediments to access to health care in their community when they read this book and to vigorously take steps to urge their state legislature and the federal government to remove those barriers. I have concluded that no change of the magnitude needed to help people with epilepsy will take place without legislation.

Criminal Justice

If people with epilepsy commit a crime they should be treated the same as anybody else. Particular problems arise when people with epilepsy are arrested because of a misinterpretation of what takes place during or immediately after a seizure. They may be unjustifiably arrested for disorderly conduct, drunkenness, creating a public disturbance, or being under the influence of drugs.

Recently, the Epilepsy Foundation of America and, separately, MINCEP Epilepsy Care and Epilepsy Education of the University of Minnesota have created training films for police officers to help mitigate this problem (see education resource list at the end of Chapter 17). A patient who has epilepsy who has been arrested may be deprived of his antiepileptic medications while in jail, resulting in further seizures. This discrimination is largely based on ignorance rather than malice, but is nonetheless harmful to the patient.

People with epilepsy are characterized as having a developmental disability and come under the protection of the "Developmental Disabilities Assistance and Bill of Rights Act." This entitles patients to help from federally mandated state developmental disability programs and from federally mandated state protection and advocacy programs.

EDUCATION

The Individuals with Disabilities Education Act provides certain protection for patients with epilepsy, particularly appropriate screening, early identification, and evaluation of children with learning problems. There is a series of complex requirements for school systems and rights for children and their parents that cannot be addressed here.

EMPLOYMENT

Federal (particularly Title V of the Rehabilitation Act) and state laws protect the patient with epilepsy from discrimination in employment. They have to be able to perform the essential functions of the job, or be able to do so with reasonable accommodation. Employers may ask job applicants whether they can perform job-related functions, but they may not inquire whether the applicant has a disability or question the severity of any disability. They may require a medical examination, but only after an offer of employment has been made, and only if the examinations are job-related, required of all employees, and are consistent with the law (Chapter 16).

SELECTED READING

1. Epilepsy Foundation of America. *The legal rights of persons with epilepsy*. 4351 Garden City Drive, Landover, MD. 301/459-3700. 1992.

Driving, Work, and Sports

16

All three of these topics are really independence issues. It doesn't help much to receive the finest medical care in the world and not have the independence to lead a fulfilling life.

Most patients with epilepsy can work in competitive employment. They have particular barriers to overcome because most employers are ignorant and many are fearful of the negative effects on their business of an employee having a seizure. The most realistic fear is that the employee will hurt himself and require coverage under Workman's Compensation Insurance. The cost of Workman's Compensation Insurance is rapidly increasing and this creates problems for many employers in many states. This does not justify discrimination against a person who is otherwise qualified to work. Recently introduced laws prevent employers from inquiring about the nature or severity of a handicap (see Chapter 15).

On the other hand, patients with epilepsy must not carry this liberation movement to an extreme. There are realistic limitations on what work people can be permitted to do if they have seizures. For example, federal law prohibits anyone who has had a loss of consciousness of any sort from

149

any cause from piloting a commercial airliner, in fact from flying any plane. They may not drive trucks in interstate commerce, and most state laws prohibit them from driving buses and school buses. Other areas where sustained, unsupervised vigilance is required may also be off limits, for example, being an air traffic controller, working on the control panel or being a safety officer in a nuclear power plant, serving as a peace officer, or operating roller coasters and similar rides in an amusement park.

Safety factors enter into less critical jobs, but often can be accommodated. Dangerous machinery such as riveting guns, punch presses, table saws, and the like may or may not be safe to operate depending on the severity of the seizures, the safeguards that can be built into the machinery, and the extent to which having a seizure will endanger others as well as the patient. Even a job as a cook in a restaurant may not be reasonable if the patient has frequent seizures and can fall into the deep fryer, for example. This still leaves thousands of types of jobs that anyone with seizures can carry out, including quite high-paying jobs such as teacher, stockbroker, lawyer, etc. Rather than trying to give an encyclopedic list of permitted and nonpermitted jobs, it is better for the physician who knows the patient's problems well to spend a few minutes with the potential employer, who knows the job requirements well, and see if they can't work out some kind of reasonable accommodation.

SPORTS

Sports are an important part of life, and certainly my patients ask about sports as often as they do about work and driving. There are certain sports in which a lapse of consciousness will undoubtedly create too great a hazard for the patient and for others. These include hang gliding, scuba diving, parachute jumping, rock climbing, bicycle and motorcycle racing, and technical mountaineering. Others tend to create an unnecessary hazard to the patient. Heavy contact sports such as football, Australian and Canadian rules, rugby, and lacrosse may be hazardous to a patient with seizures. Ice hockey is becoming a heavy contact sport and should be avoided at the highly competitive level.

It is more difficult to pass judgment on archery, skeet shooting, target shooting, javelin throwing, the discus, and other sports in which a projectile is used. Patients with prolonged automatisms probably should not participate in these sports. Patients with absence attacks or simple GTCs (generalized tonic-clonic seizures) probably can. Skiing, both cross country and downhill, may be hazardous with certain kinds of seizures, yet excellent exercise for patients with other kinds of seizures.

Swimming is a particularly difficult problem. It is good exercise, readily available, and commonly provided as recreation to children in summer camp. Drowning is an unusually common form of death for people with seizures. Patients can drown in 3 inches of water in the bathtub as easily as in 30 feet of water in a lake. For patients with infrequent seizures, swimming with a buddy system is usually safe, especially if the lifeguard has been alerted. Nonetheless, it is more hazardous for patients with epilepsy than for those who don't have seizures. Accidents can and have happened and resuscitation is not always possible (see Table 16.1).

RISKS IN LIFE

Life is inherently dangerous. We are all subject to unexpected accidents. Life in some parts of the world is more hazardous than in others. Life in certain times in history has been more hazardous than others. One must adopt a balanced attitude toward risk and not deprive a child or young adult with epilepsy from wholesome activity just because the risk is slightly higher. We cannot protect our loved ones from every hazard in this world.

Table 16.1   *Relative risk of sports for people with seizures**

Low Risk, Minimal or No Supervision

Aerobics	Discus
Badminton	Fencing
Baseball (H)	Field Hockey (H)
Bowling	Golf
Cricket	High Jump
Croquet	Hiking
Cross-Country Skiing	Jogging
(no long, steep hills)	Long Jump
Curling	Ping Pong
Dancing	Running
(all types except	Soccer (H)
break dancing)	Softball (H)

Moderate Risk, Low to Moderate Supervision

Archery	Parallel Bars (H—low only)
Basketball (H)	Rollerblading (H)
Bicycling (H)	Roller-skating (H)
Bobsledding (H)	Rugby (H)
Canoeing (S)	Sailing (S—no one-person boats)
Diving (S—low board only)	Sledding (H)
Downhill Skiing (H)	Snorkeling (S)
Fishing	Tennis
Football (H)	Snowmobiling (H—if okay to drive)
Horse (H)	Swimming (S)
Horseback Riding (H)	Tumbling
Hunting	Volleyball
Ice Hockey (H)	Wrestling
Ice Skating (H)	Waterskiing (S)
Orienteering	

**High Risk, Generally Prohibited Unless Seizure Free
and Off Medicine for 5 Years**

Boxing (prohibited at all times)	Hang Gliding
Mountain Climbing	Bungee Jumping
Rock Climbing	Surfing
Sky Diving	Wind Surfing
Scuba Diving	

---

*In general, rigorous physical activity is to be encouraged. The general principle is to avoid situations where a sudden loss of consciousness can hurt the patient or an innocent bystander.

H: must wear a helmet. S: Swim precautions: buddy system as well as lifeguard and/or life preserver.

DRIVING

Inability to drive is perhaps the greatest restriction in the life of most people with epilepsy. Few people can live a normal life in nearly all the United States without a driver's license and access to a car. There are a few cities with adequate public transportation and recreational resources so that a car isn't necessary, but these opportunities are present for only a fraction of the population. As a result, patients with epilepsy find themselves frustrated and often pressure their physician to stretch the law, tell a white lie, or overlook an obvious hazard.

It is both the law and common sense that people who are at high risk for loss of consciousness, and hence losing control of an automobile, should not be permitted to drive. The issue is whether the specific patient in your examining room presents such a risk. The accompanying table (Table 16.2) lists the regulations of the 50 states and the District of Columbia at the time of writing. These laws change with each session of the state legislature. Consult the Epilepsy Foundation of America for an up-to-date list. They do a valuable public service by updating this table on a regular basis.

From a purely medical point of view there are some considerations to guide the physician. Patients who have a sudden loss of consciousness without warning are clearly at greater risk for accidents than someone who has a prolonged aura that does not affect consciousness or has only a simple partial seizure without motor dysfunction. Patients whose seizures are only nocturnal are at lesser risk than those whose seizures may occur at any time of the day or night.

Although physicians cannot change the law, it is important to note that epilepsy is no more likely to create frequent automobile accidents (on a population basis) than diabetes, heart disease, or mental disorders, and substantially less likely to cause trouble than alcoholism and drug abuse (see attached driving and epilepsy chart).

Table 16.2 *Driving and epilepsy*

State	Seizure -Free Period	Periodic Medical Updates Required After Licensing	Doctors Required to Report Epilepsy	DMV Appeal of License Denial*
Alabama	1 year	Annually for 10 years from date of last seizure	No	Within 10 days
Alaska	6 months	At discretion of Department of Motor Vehicles	No	Within 15 days
Arizona	3 months, with exceptions	At discretion of Motor Vehicle Division	No	Within 15 days
Arkansas	1 year	At discretion of Department of Motor Vehicles	No	Within 20 days
California	3, 6 or 12 months with exceptions	As above	Yes	Within 10 days
Colorado	No set seizure-free period	As above	No	Yes
Connecticut	No set seizure-free period	As above	No	Yes
Delaware	No set seizure-free period	Annually	Yes	Yes
District of Columbia	1 year, with exceptions	Annually until 5 years seizure-free	No	Within 5 days
Florida	6 months with exceptions	At discretion of Medical Advisory Board	No	Yes
Georgia	1 year. Less if only nocturnal seizures	At discretion of Department of Motor Vehicles	No	Within 15 days
Hawaii	1 year, with exceptions	At discretion of Department of Motor Vehicles	No	Yes

This chart was developed for information purposes by the Epilepsy Foundation of America's Legal Advocacy Department and reflects data available as of November 1993. Information is subject to change. This chart is not a substitute for legal advice. For further information, consult your state Department of Motor Vehicles.

**Time frames within which one must request an administrative review or hearing are given when known. Every state allows for appeal of license denial through the courts.*

***Note: Non-driver I.D. cards are available in every state.*

Table 16.2 *Driving and epilepsy (continued)*

State	Seizure-Free Period	Periodic Medical Updates Required After Licensing	Doctors Required to Report Epilepsy	DMV Appeal of License Denial*
Idaho	1 year, 6 months with strong recommendation from doctor	Annually	No	Any time
Illinois	No set seizure-free period	At discretion of Medical Advisory Board	No	Yes
Indiana	No set seizure-free period	As above	No	Yes
Iowa	6 months. Less if seizures nocturnal	After first 6 months, then at renewal	No	Within 30 days
Kansas	6 months	Annually, until 3 years seizure-free	No	Within 30 days
Kentucky	90 days	On renewal	No	Within 20 days
Louisiana	1 year, with exceptions	At discretion of Department of Motor Vehicles	No	No
Maine	6 months or longer	As above	No	Yes
Maryland	90 days	As above	No	Within 15 days
Massachusetts	6 months	At discretion of Medical Advisory Board	No	Within 14 days
Michigan	6 months. Less at discretion of department	At discretion of Medical Advisory Board	No	Within 14 days
Minnesota	6 months, with exceptions	Every 6 months until 1 year seizure-free; then annually for 4 yrs.; then every 4 yrs.	No	Yes
Mississippi	1 year	At discretion of Medical Advisory Board	No	No
Missouri	1 year	At license renewal	No	No

Table 16.2 *Driving and epilepsy (continued)*

State	Seizure -Free Period	Periodic Medical Updates Required After Licensing	Doctors Required to Report Epilepsy	DMV Appeal of License Denial*
Montana	6 months	No	No	Yes
Nebraska	1 year, with exceptions	No	No	Yes
Nevada	3 months, with exceptions	Annually	Yes	Within 30 days
New Hampshire	1 year, less at discretion of department	No	No	Within 30 days
New Jersey	1 year, less with recommendation of Neurological Disorder Committee	Every 6 months for 2 years, thereafter annually	Yes	Within 10 days
New Mexico	1 year	At discretion of Medical Advisory Board	No	Within 20 days
New York	1 year, with exceptions	At discretion of Department of Motor Vehicles	No	Within 30 days
North Carolina	1 year with exceptions	Annually, less at discretion of Department of Motor Vehicles	No	Within 10 days
North Dakota	1 year. Restricted licenses available after 6 months	Annually for at least 5 years	No	Within 10 days
Ohio	No set seizure-free period	Every 6 months or 1 year until seizure-free 5 years	No	Within 30 days
Oklahoma	1 year, with exceptions	At discretion of Department of Public Safety	No	Yes
Oregon	6 months, with exceptions	Every 6 or 12 months until at least 2 years seizure-free	Yes	Within 20 days
Pennsylvania	6 months, with exceptions	At discretion of Medical Advisory Board	Yes	Yes

Table 16.2 *Driving and epilepsy (continued)*

State	Seizure-Free Period	Periodic Medical Updates Required After Licensing	Doctors Required to Report Epilepsy	DMV Appeal of License Denial*
Puerto Rico	No set seizure-free period	As above	No	Within 20 days
Rhode Island	18 months; less at discretion of Department of Transportation	As above	No	Within 10 days
South Carolina	6 months	Every 6 months	No	Within 10 days
South Dakota	12 months. Less with doctor's recommendation	Every 6 months until 1 year seizure-free	No	No
Tennessee	6 months	At discretion of Medical Advisory Board	No	Within 20 days
Texas	6 months with doctor's recommendation, with exceptions	At discretion of Medical Advisory Board	No	No
Utah	3 months	Every 6 months until 1 year seizure-free	No	Within 10 days
Vermont	24 months, or 6 months with doctor's recommendation	Every 6 months until 2 years seizure-free	No	Within 10 days
Virginia	6 months, with exceptions	At discretion of Medical Advisory Board	No	Yes
Washington	6 months	As above	No	Anytime
West Virginia	1 year, with exceptions	As above	No	Within 10 days
Wisconsin	3 months	At discretion of Department of Motor Vehicles	No	Yes
Wyoming	1 year, with exceptions	Annually, until seizure-free 2 years, thereafter upon license renewal	No	Within 20 days

SELECTED READING

1. Corbitt RW. Epileptics and contact sports. *JAMA* 1974; 229: 820–821.

17   # Community Resources

Patients with epilepsy need help with advocacy, information, social services and financial aid, and counseling. A book of this sort cannot possibly list every community agency in every city in the country, but what follows is a brief guide on how to find out what is available in your community.

PATIENT ADVOCACY AND PATIENT EDUCATIONAL MATERIALS

The Epilepsy Foundation of America (EFA) provides a national WATS line to help physicians and their patients with this kind of information. Simply call one of the numbers below and they will help you find a local group for your patients:

Physicians can call 1-800-EFA-4050
Patients can call 1-800 EFA-1000
4351 Garden City Drive
Landover, Maryland 20788

EFA can also provide information about their training and placement service (TAPS) for patients who need help finding a job.

For information about specialized epilepsy centers, contact the National Association of Comprehensive Epilepsy Centers, 5775 Wayzata Blvd., Minneapolis, MN 55416; (612) 525-4526.

SOCIAL SERVICE NEEDS, FINANCIAL ASSISTANCE, AND FAMILY COUNSELING

Most communities have a family service agency of some sort, usually several. Church-supported agencies include Catholic Charities, Jewish Family Service, Lutheran Aid Society, and numerous other protestant groups. Nondenominational community organizations are also widely available.

Hospitals usually have a social service department and provide a ready source of reference to community agencies. Hospital social workers collaborate with them all the time.

PSYCHOLOGICAL COUNSELING

There are many psychiatrists and psychologists in private practice. Community mental health centers and other mental health clinics are widely distributed. Again, the hospital social service department or a community social service agency will know what is available in your community.

VOCATIONAL PLACEMENT

The federal government provides help through the Division of Vocational Rehabilitation or a similar organization in every state. The state Developmental Disabilities Agency also can be consulted if there are problems with hiring and affirmative action.

Not every physician's office will have its own social worker or psychologist, but every physician and physician's office nurse should be familiar with the problems that patients with epilepsy have and be able to guide them to appropriate local help.

<table><tr><td>18</td><td># Clinical Vignettes</td></tr></table>

PARTIAL SEIZURES

Simple Partial Seizures

Arthur G. consulted his family physician, Dr. White. He was frightened. The day before, while driving his car on the freeway, his left hand suddenly lifted off the steering wheel and began to shake rhythmically. Try as he might, he could not control it. Fortunately, he did not lose consciousness and pulled the car over to the side of the highway safely. By the time he had parked the car, everything was back to normal. In response to Dr. White's questions, Mr. G. told of having received a shrapnel wound in the right frontal lobe while on active duty in Vietnam 3 years previously. An operation was performed within a few hours of the injury, and he had been discharged from the Army with no apparent sequelae. Dr. White knew that the onset of a partial seizure in a young adult often meant an underlying brain tumor or arteriovenous malformation. However, the site of Mr. G.'s wound coincided with the site of this focal motor seizure that could be localized purely on a clinical basis; an MRI scan revealed no evidence of a new process.

Mr. G. had been taking phenytoin (300 mg/day) for 2 years after the wound, but his physician had stopped the drug 6 months before the seizure. Dr. White reinstituted phenytoin and found that 300 mg/day gave Mr. G. a serum level of 9 g/ml. Increasing the dosage to 330 mg/day brought Mr. G. to a serum phenytoin level of 14 g/ml, which satisfied Dr. White. Mr. G. had no further seizures. At Dr. White's suggestion, Mr. G. did not drive an automobile until his drug level was satisfactory. Dr. White concluded that phenytoin successfully suppressed Mr. G.'s seizures, and that this episode was brought about by his following the physician's recommendation to stop anticonvulsant treatment.

Anticonvulsants will suppress seizures but not cure them. It is standard practice to stop anticonvulsants 2 or 3 years after a head injury, but some patients may need to take the medicine for a prolonged period, even for a lifetime. This is the situation in Mr. G.'s case. Because the seizures were well suppressed with adequate doses of phenytoin, there was no reason for Mr. G. to refrain from driving an automobile for a year once an adequate serum phenytoin level had been reached.

Complex Partial Seizures

An 18-year-old girl, Mary T., was referred to Dr. Black, a neurologist. She had been under the care of physicians in another state but had recently moved, with her parents, when her father had accepted a new job. Her new family physician had referred her to Dr. Black because Mary had told him that she was continuing to have two to three seizures a year even though she had been seen by a family doctor and a neurologist in her previous home state. Her parents complained that she was emotionally unstable and lacked "pep."

Her parents had first become aware of Mary's seizures when she was 15 years of age. They had received a telephone call from school stating that Mary had had a strange episode and suggesting that she see the family doctor. According to the teacher, Mary had suddenly begun to raise and lower the tilting top on her desk in class. This was disruptive of classroom activities. When asked to stop, Mary looked blankly at the teacher and began to fumble with the buttons on her sweater. The teacher walked toward Mary to see what was wrong, but Mary put her arms out in front of her as if to ward off the teacher. She then stood up and began to wander aimlessly about the room. In a few minutes she stopped, looked around in a puzzled manner, went back to her desk, put her head down, and took a brief nap.

Mary was terribly embarrassed by this episode. No one in class really told her what she had done, yet she knew she had somehow behaved in a peculiar fashion. She was reluctant to return to school, and it was only with a great effort on the part of her parents, her family doctor, and the strong support of her teachers that Mary found the courage to go back to school.

As her new neurologist talked with Mary and her parents, it became evident that for several months before this episode Mary had had brief lapses when she seemed to lose track of what was going on. Her parents kidded her about being absentminded, and her usual "A" for conduct and cooperation in class had dropped to "C." Her former doctors had started Mary on phenobarbital (4 mg/kg). This treatment had led to a reduction of both the smaller lapses and the larger seizures, so that Mary had experienced only three episodes in the past year. Although her physicians had been satisfied with that degree of seizure control, Mary felt dopey all day long and suffered constant anxiety about the possibility of having another seizure in front of her schoolmates. She was also concerned about whether she would be permitted to take driver's training and get her driver's license.

Dr. Black ordered an electroencephalogram (EEG), which revealed frequent sharp-wave discharges from the right temporal lobe. Further questioning of the parents revealed that Mary had been born precipitously. She was a first child, yet labor had lasted only 45 min. Because of the focal nature of her seizures and EEG, further studies were ordered. The magnetic resonance imaging (MRI) scan was normal, and neuropsychological studies, including special nondominant temporal lobe batteries, revealed evidence of mild right temporal lobe dysfunction. Carbamazepine was started at a dose of 200 mg twice a day and was gradually increased until the plasma level reached 6 g/ml. Phenobarbital was tapered off over a period of 3 months. Mary was much brighter and less irritable once the phenobarbital was stopped. On this regimen, she has had no further partial complex seizures.

Mary was encouraged to take the classroom portion of driver's education. She will be eligible to take behind-the-wheel training as soon as she has been seizure free for 6 months. Dr. Black explained to Mary in detail about her seizures and the cause of her brain damage. If the seizures recur she will be considered for epilepsy surgery. Her parents report that her psychological attitude has improved now that she has a better understanding of her condition and is no longer so drowsy. Before seeing Dr. Black, Mary had been feeling helpless and hopeless. She is now beginning to make plans for further education and to talk about a career.

Partial Seizures Evolving to Generalized Tonic-Clonic Convulsions

Benjamin H., a 47-year-old truck driver, consulted his family physician after having a generalized tonic-clonic seizure. His wife said that early one Monday morning she heard a noise and found him beside the bed with his arms and legs extended and his back arched. The position was followed by a series of brief relaxations and subsequent tonic extension in a rhythmic fashion. The seizure lasted about 90 sec, and Mr. H. then fell into a deep sleep from which he did not waken for more than an hour.

Mr. H. has a history of moderately heavy drinking, but had never missed work because of alcoholism and had no history of arrests for drunken driving. He had been up late the preceding Friday and Saturday nights playing poker and drinking, but had spent Sunday playing ball with his oldest boy and doing yard work.

His family doctor thought this episode might have been an alcohol withdrawal seizure and told Mr. H. to stop drinking. His brief physical and neurological examinations showed no abnormalities, and an EEG revealed nonspecific slow activity. Mr. H. reduced his drinking substantially, although he did have an occasional social drink. Nonetheless, a second generalized tonic-clonic seizure occurred about 2 months later.

His family doctor told Mr. H. to stop driving and prescribed phenytoin (300 mg/day). This dosage produced a serum phenytoin level of 12 g/ml. Mr. H. pointed out that he could not earn a living if he could not drive. While he and his doctor were wrestling with the significance of this problem, he had a third seizure despite a phenytoin level of 14 g/ml. At this point, the family doctor referred Mr. H. to a neurologist. The neurologist was concerned about the sudden onset of generalized seizures in a middle-aged man for no apparent cause. His neurological examination revealed minimal drift in the left arm and some loss in swing of the left arm when Mr. H. walked.

An EEG showed focal slow activity in the right frontal area interictally, and a brief electrographic seizure arising focally in that area was observed. A CT scan was obtained that the x-ray department reported as probably normal, although a questionable area of increased radiolucency was noted in the right frontal area. An MRI revealed a Grade III astrocytoma. The focal nature of Mr. H.'s seizures was missed clinically because it was buried in the rapid onset of the generalized seizure. It was only because an EEG examination was taking place during an attack that the focal component was recognized.

GENERALIZED SEIZURES

Absence Seizures

The school called Mrs. B. to report that her daughter, Joan, was apparently inattentive in her first grade class. A substitute teacher reported that Joan would sometimes stare at her blankly and blink her eyes for a few seconds at a time. She did not respond to her name when this happened.

Mrs. B. immediately consulted Dr. White, her family physician. She told Dr. White that a similar event had occurred to her when she was a child and that Joan's older brother, Roger, had also had similar difficulty. Dr. White asked Joan to hyperventilate, and after 1 min of deep breathing, Joan began to blink her eyes and stare and was unresponsive. An EEG confirmed the diagnosis of absence attacks, revealing bilaterally synchronous and symmetrical 3/sec spikes and slow waves, maximal in the frontal region. Roger's EEG revealed similar activity, but the mother's EEG was normal. Dr. White concluded that he was dealing with a simple case of familial absence seizures, and prescribed ethosuximide (250 mg twice a day). This therapy brought about an immediate halt to the seizures. Although some EEG discharges were still present, hyperventilation no longer produced clinical attacks. Since neither the mother nor Roger were having clinical seizures, Dr. White elected not to treat them. He told Mrs. B. that had there been a history of generalized tonic-clonic seizures in the family he would have also prescribed phenytoin for Joan because the two types of seizures often go together. However, he and the mother elected to take the risk of a possible generalized tonic-clonic seizure to avoid unnecessarily prescribing a second antiepileptic medicine.

BILATERAL CLONIC SEIZURES WITH FEVER

Mrs. S. rushed her 2-year-old son, James, to the emergency room of the local hospital. The boy had a temperature of 105°F for unknown reasons. On arrival in the emergency room, the child began to have rhythmic shaking of all extremities with a disturbance of normal breathing. The seizures lasted for only 30 sec or so and were repeated about every 15 min for about an hour. The child's temperature was rapidly brought down by a combination of aspirin and body cooling. The appearance of a typical rash the next day confirmed the diagnosis of roseola. Mrs. S. was worried about the seizures, but it became clear to the pediatrician that this was the third child in the family to have similar episodes with high fever. Neither of the first two had developed epilepsy. Mrs. S. was reassured and told that no treatment was necessary. Had the seizures been unduly sustained, indicating poor inhibitory mechanisms at work in the child's brain, or had there been a family history of epilepsy, the physician might well have elected to treat the child prophylactically until he had passed the age of 5 years.

BREATH-HOLDING SPELLS

Mrs. P. consulted a pediatric neurologist at the suggestion of her family doctor. Her 3-year-old son, Frank, had had fetal distress and neonatal seizures. He spent the first 3 weeks of life in a neonatal intensive care unit. However, he had had no seizures since and his milestones were coming along normally. Recently, Mrs. P. had noted two episodes that frightened her. Frank had been running across the living room floor attempting to catch the family puppy. He tripped and fell, striking his chin. He burst into tears, seemed to have difficulty breathing, got blue around the lips, stiffened all over, and then shook slightly. This lasted less than a minute. After this episode, he cried weakly and seemed to be very tired. Two weeks later, the boy attempted to touch the top of the stove. Mrs. P. slapped his hand and told him "no" in a sharp voice. The child looked at her with wide eyes. His jaw dropped open and he started to scream. His eyes rolled back, he stopped breathing, and had what appeared to be a brief convulsion.

The family doctor suggested that she consult a pediatric neurologist because he knew of the difficulty encountered in separating breath-holding spells from tonic or myoclonic seizures. He was particularly concerned because of the child's history of genuine seizures during infancy. Discussion between Mrs. P. and the neurologist could not produce any history of episodes occurring spontaneously. There had been only two episodes, and both of these had occurred in response to environmental stress. The neurological examination showed no abnormalities. EEG examinations, including a sleep tracing, did not reveal any seizure activity.

The consulting neurologist concluded that the child was probably having simple breath-holding spells and recommended against treatment with anticonvulsants. Mrs. P. was told to return if the episodes became more of a problem or something new developed.

MIXED SEIZURES

Sally T. was wearing out her welcome in the offices of the many physicians that she and her family and various social agencies had consulted. At the age of 29, she was living in a board and care home and working at a sheltered workshop. When MINCEP Epilepsy Care first opened its comprehensive epilepsy program, everyone concerned agreed that if Sally were to be helped it would be at MINCEP.

At the time of the admission interview, things did not look too hopeful. Sally was a 29-year-old woman of borderline intelligence who had never held a job in the competitive world. Her behavior was highly dependent. She was having an average of 11 seizures a week. The descriptions of the seizures were varied and confusing, and some of the attacks were even thought to be hysterical seizures.

On admission, she had no physical abnormalities except obesity and poor skin condition. Her neurological examination also showed no abnormalities. Psychological evaluation revealed a slightly elevated HYS score on the Minnesota Multiphasic Personality Inventory (MMPI) and an IQ of 85 on the Wechsler Adult Intelligence Scale (WAIS), but planning skills were within the normal range.

Her antiepileptic medicines were gradually withdrawn except for phenytoin (360 mg/day), which provided a plasma level of 18 g/ml. Prolonged video/EEG monitoring revealed that Sally had three kinds of spells:

1. Brief episodes of confusion with semipurposeful movements and amnesia for the event. These spells generally lasted 3 to 5 sec and were accompanied by rhythmic sharp-wave discharges in the right temporal lobe

2. Brief sudden loss of muscle tone during which she fell to the floor and lost consciousness. The EEG consisted of bilaterally synchronous high-voltage 3/sec bursts intermixed with spike activity. On several occasions, she bit her tongue or lacerated her chin. The nursing staff determined it would be in her best interest to wear a hockey helmet while these episodes continued

3. Prolonged episodes of crying and moaning with alternate jerking of the left and right arm and kicking of both legs. These episodes were occasionally accompanied by excess

salivation but no incontinence. They were not accompanied by any definite EEG changes, and seemed to be stimulated by environmental frustrations

A CT scan revealed some scattered atrophy in the frontal and temporal lobes bilaterally, presumably secondary to childhood encephalitis.

It was determined that Sally had three types of seizures. She had complex partial seizures arising in the right temporal lobe, she had generalized atonic drop attacks of multifocal origin, and she also had psychogenic seizures mimicking generalized tonic-clonic seizures. No true generalized tonic-clonic seizures were observed, but it was noted that she had been protected with phenytoin.

Carbamazepine in doses that produced a serum level of 5 g/ml completely controlled the complex partial seizures. She continued to have the drop attacks, but these were brought under control with valproic acid at a serum level of 90 g/ml 1 hr after the dose.

Sally noticed increased appetite. This was a particular management problem because she was already obese. Once the complex partial seizures and drop attacks had been brought under control, phenytoin was gradually discontinued. Over several months, Sally noted an improvement in her skin condition.

The doctors explained to Sally that she had three types of seizures. Two were genuine brain events that could be treated with anticonvulsants, and one was her way of responding to stress in the environment. Intense individual counseling aimed at teaching better coping mechanisms was undertaken. Other patients helped her to distinguish between the real seizures and the psychogenic attacks. During semiweekly group sessions, she confronted the troubles she was creating for herself with inappropriate behavior.

With the genuine seizures under good control, and a clearer understanding of her psychogenic seizures, the social agencies and Sally's family were more effective in shaping her behavior. Gradually, over the course of the next year, the psychogenic seizures were replaced with more appropriate coping mechanisms, and Sally was able to obtain employment in a factory. A year later, she and another employee decided to room together, and for the first time in her life, this young woman was living independently in the community. She keeps her medical appointments and has been compliant in taking her anticonvulsant medications.

JUVENILE MYOCLONIC EPILEPSY

Joan's mother became exasperated with her 17-year-old daughter. This otherwise healthy and intelligent young woman suddenly seemed to be behaving bizarrely. When she would get up to go to school in the morning her hairbrush would go flying through the air. On one occasion it cracked the mirror. Subsequently, Joan developed what appeared to be an absence or brief complex partial seizure. Before Joan's mother recognized what was going on, Joan had a generalized tonic-clonic seizure. By this time, everyone in the family was greatly alarmed and her family consulted Dr. Smith. Dr. Smith, a family practitioner, was puzzled why something like this should appear out of the blue in his otherwise healthy patient. Neither he nor the family associated the hairbrush episodes with the generalized tonic-clonic seizure. Dr. Smith prescribed phenytoin for the generalized tonic-clonic seizure. To his surprise, Joan continued to have seizures and the family became increasingly alarmed.

Dr. Smith referred Joan to a neurologist, who managed to put all the pieces together. He diagnosed Joan as having juvenile myoclonic epilepsy (JME, also called Janz syndrome) and prescribed Depakote instead. Joan's seizures immediately ceased. The neurologist had warned Joan about the possibility of increased appetite and loss of hair with the use of Depakote. She was a self-contained young woman, who immediately put herself on a controlled diet.

She has suffered no untoward side effects and has graduated from college.

Joan may be able to stop her Depakote when she gets a bit older, but many patients with JME will take small doses of valproic acid for many years.

HIPPOCAMPAL SCLEROSIS

George developed complex partial seizures at the age of 4 years. These were treated by his family doctor in rural Oklahoma with phenobarbital. Although the seizures were brought under reasonable control, George felt groggy, became irritable, and misbehaved. His family doctor switched him to Dilantin with excellent results and complete seizure control without side effects. However, by the time George was 14 years old, the seizures recurred, and despite increasing doses of Dilantin and a trial on Tegretol, the seizures continued to be a major problem. By this time, George and his family were feeling desperate, and they found their way to MINCEP Epilepsy Care in Minneapolis. The doctors at MINCEP were particularly alerted by the fact that the seizures had begun at an early age, were initially controlled, and had now become more severe. An MRI with thin cuts carefully aligned perpendicular to the plane of the temporal lobe revealed a slightly atrophic hippocampus in the right temporal lobe. Video/EEGs revealed consistent interictal sharp-waves from the mesial portion of the right temporal lobe, and several seizures were observed on video/EEG. These were typical of George's seizures at home with a brief stare and automatism. The ictal events all began before the behavioral events, and also arose in the mesial portion of the right temporal lobe. Neuropsychological studies revealed deficits in the functioning of the mesial portion of the right temporal lobe; otherwise the patient was of normal intelligence and fully intact. Because major antiepileptic drugs had failed the patient and he had the classic syndrome of mesial temporal sclerosis, it was elected to operate to perform a right anterior temporal lobectomy rather than to procrastinate. The operation was uneventful, and George has been seizure free ever since. He continues on small doses of Tegretol as a precaution. He has a small field defect that is clinically not significant, as the result of sectioning Meyer's loop of the visual radiation, which swings anteriorly through the mesial portion of the temporal lobe, but no additional deficits appeared on his neuropsychological exam. Now that George is seizure free he is driving a car and is looking forward to a full and fulfilling life.

EXTRATEMPORAL COMPLEX PARTIAL SEIZURES

John W. was a successful mechanical engineer from Denmark. At the age of 35 he began to develop seizures in which there were focal motor problems in the right arm and arrest of behavior. On occasion there were adversive movements of the eyes to the right. MRI studies revealed an atrophic area surrounding an arteriovenous malformation in the left frontal lobe anterior but adjacent to the motor strip. The seizures could not be controlled even with very high doses of antiepileptic drugs and his performance as an engineer was suffering from the sedative effects of his medicine. He was referred by the University Hospital in Copenhagen to MINCEP Epilepsy Care to see if he might possibly be a candidate for surgery. Because the seizures were intractable, he was suffering from toxicity, and there was a clearly identifiable anatomic lesion, it was decided to proceed with surgery. A subdural electrode array (grid) was placed over the area of the lesion and the motor and speech areas of the left frontal lobe. Video/EEG recording revealed stereotypical seizures occurring in an area of the brain that was adjacent to but not congruous with either motor strip or speech area. The motor strip and the speech area were outlined by stimulation through the electrodes, and a functional cortical map was prepared. A resection was designed that would remove the epileptogenic area without invading the two areas of vital cortex. This was carried out, and the patient has been seizure free on small doses of Tegretol ever since.

DROP ATTACKS

Elizabeth W. was a 17-year-old living in Auckland, New Zealand. She had suffered some ill-defined birth injury and was left with mild mental retardation and a little clumsiness. More significantly, she had frequent tonic seizures of the Salaaem type, which caused her to drop to the floor and injure herself. She had lacerated her scalp on several occasions, had knocked out some teeth, and had broken a bone. Her parents brought her to MINCEP Epilepsy Care to see what could be done medically or surgically to help her. She had been tried on high doses of all the antiepileptic drugs including Depakote, Klonopin, and Mogadon, and none of these had helped her. Her video/EEG showed a bilateral fast pattern associated with the seizures. She was taken to the operating room and an anterior two-thirds section of the corpus callosum was carried out. This resulted in immediate reduction of frequency and severity of her drop attacks. Two years later her family reported that she no longer had daily attacks. She was having one or two attacks a month, but rather than dropping precipitously to the floor she tended to collapse in a "more ladylike swoon." Now that her seizures were under much improved control, she had obtained competitive employment as a chambermaid in a downtown hotel, was living independently of her family in a boardinghouse, and was developing a social life. She continues on small doses of Depakote, however.

Appendix

1. PATIENT'S DIARY

Fill out each morning and bring this form with you when you see the doctor.

Date:

	Monday		Tuesday		Wednesday		Thursday		Friday		Saturday		Sunday	
	Time Taken		Time Taken		Time Taken		Time Taken		Time Taken		Time Taken		Time Taken	
Drugs Rx	#1	#2	#1	#2	#1	#2	#1	#2	#1	#2	#1	#2	#1	#2
	____am	____am	____am	____am	____am	____am	____am	____am	____am	____am	____am	____am	____am	____am
#1: ______	____	____	____	____	____	____	____	____	____	____	____	____	____	____
	____	____	____	____	____	____	____	____	____	____	____	____	____	____
#2: ______	____pm	____pm	____pm	____pm	____pm	____pm	____pm	____pm	____pm	____pm	____pm	____pm	____pm	____pm
Seizure Type 1	0, <1, 1-2, 3-5, ____		0, <1, 1-2, 3-5, ____		0, <1, 1-2, 3-5, ____		0, <1, 1-2, 3-5, ____		0, <1, 1-2, 3-5, ____		0, <1, 1-2, 3-5, ____		0, <1, 1-2, 3-5, __	
Describe:														
	Time: ______		Time: ______		Time: ______		Time: ______		Time: ______		Time: ______		Time: ______	
Seizure Type 2	0, <1, 1-2, 3-5, ____		0, <1, 1-2, 3-5, ____		0, <1, 1-2, 3-5, ____		0, <1, 1-2, 3-5, ____		0, <1, 1-2, 3-5, ____		0, <1, 1-2, 3-5, ____		0, <1, 1-2, 3-5, __	
Describe:														
	Time: ______		Time: ______		Time: ______		Time: ______		Time: ______		Time: ______		Time: ______	
Seizure Type 3	0, <1, 1-2, 3-5, ____		0, <1, 1-2, 3-5, ____		0, <1, 1-2, 3-5, ____		0, <1, 1-2, 3-5, ____		0, <1, 1-2, 3-5, ____		0, <1, 1-2, 3-5, ____		0, <1, 1-2, 3-5, __	
Describe:														
	Time: ______		Time: ______		Time: ______		Time: ______		Time: ______		Time: ______		Time: ______	

Comments:

2. PHYSICIAN'S DIARY

Drug name	Date:		Date:		Date:		Date:	
	Dose (mg/day)	Serum level (μg/ml)	Dose (mg/day)	Serum level (μg/ml)	Dose (mg/day)	Serum level (μg/ml)	Dose (mg/day)	Serum level (μg/ml)
Drug 1								
Drug 2								
Drug 3								
Drug 4								

	No. of seizures/week	No. of seizures/week	No. of seizures/week	No. of seizures/week
Seizure type 1 Describe:	0,<1, 1–2, 3–5,____ Time of day:____	0,<1, 1–2, 3–5,____ Time of day:____	0,<1, 1–2, 3–5,____ Time of day:____	0,<1, 1–2, 3–5,____ Time of day:____
Seizure type 2 Describe:	0,<1, 1–2, 3–5,____ Time of day:____	0,<1, 1–2, 3–5,____ Time of day:____	0,<1, 1–2, 3–5,____ Time of day:____	0,<1, 1–2, 3–5,____ Time of day:____
Seizure type 3 Describe:	0,<1, 1–2, 3–5,____ Time of day:____	0,<1, 1–2, 3–5,____ Time of day:____	0,<1, 1–2, 3–5,____ Time of day:____	0,<1, 1–2, 3–5,____ Time of day:____
Toxicity	Time of day:____	Time of day:____	Time of day:____	Time of day:____

Comments:

3. FIRST AID FOR EPILEPSY

Generalized Tonic-Clonic Seizures

During the seizure: The person may fall, become stiff and make jerking movements. The person's complexion may become pale or bluish.

- DO help the person lie down and put something soft under the head.
- DO remove any eyeglasses and loosen any tight clothing.
- DO clear the area of sharp or hard objects.
- DO NOT force anything into the person's mouth.
- DO NOT try to restrain the person. You cannot stop the seizure.

After the seizure: The person may awaken confused and disoriented.

- DO turn the person to one side to allow saliva to drain from the mouth.
- DO arrange for someone to stay nearby until the person is fully awake.
- DO NOT offer the person any food or drink

Complex Partial Seizures

During the seizure: The person may have a glassy stare; give no response or an inappropriate response when questioned; sit, stand, or walk aimlessly; make lip-smacking or chewing motions; fidget or remove clothes; appear to be drunk, drugged, or even psychotic.

- DO try to remove harmful objects from the person's pathway or coax the person away from them.

- DO NOT try to stop or restrain the person.
- DO NOT agitate the person.
- DO NOT approach the person if you are alone and the person appears to be angry or aggressive. This is very unusual.

After the seizure: The person may be confused or disoriented after regaining consciousness and should not be left alone until fully alert.

Calling for Help

Call 911 or the local police **if** . . .

- The person does not start breathing within 1 minute after the seizure ends (begin mouth-to-mouth resuscitation).
- A generalized tonic-clonic seizure lasts more than 2 minutes.
- The person has one seizure right after another.
- The person is injured.
- The person requests an ambulance.

4. POSITIONING OF PATIENT WITH GENERALIZED TONIC-CLONIC SEIZURES

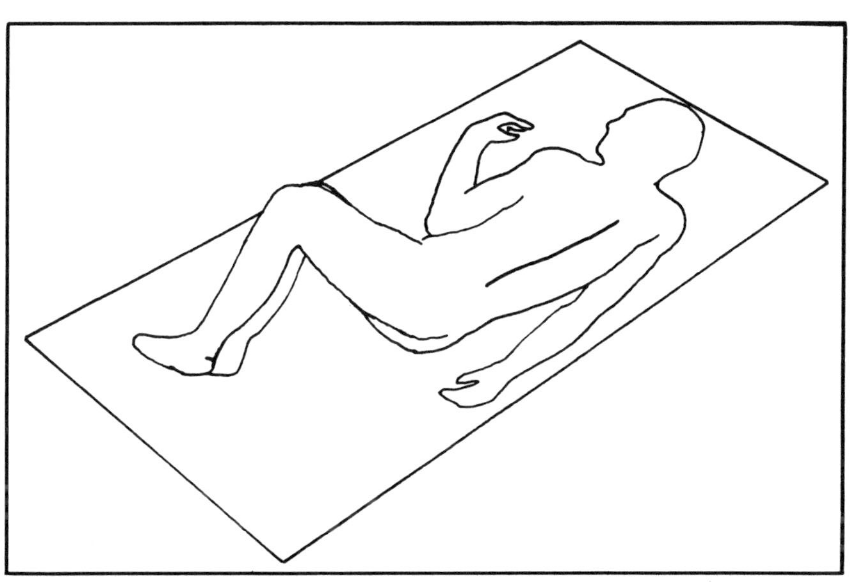

5. ANECDOTAL RECORD
FOR THE STUDENT WITH EPILEPSY

Student's name_______________________________________

Date of Seizure _______________ Time of Seizure__________

What was the student's behavior before the seizure (precipitating events, if any?) ______________________________

____

____

____

What was the student's behavior during the seizure (sides and parts of the body involved during the seizure, e.g., incontinence, sequential order of movements)? ___________

____

____

____

How long did the seizure last? _________________________

How long was the patient confused after the seizure? ____

____

Describe any injuries from the seizure___________________

____

____

____

Teacher's name (print)
and telephone number _________________ Date________

6. INFORMATION FORM
FOR THE STUDENT WITH EPILEPSY

Student's Name _______________ Birth Date ______ Sex __

Parent's Name______________ Home Phone ___________

Address ____

Physicians's Name_____________________________________

Types of Seizures ____________________________________

Receiving Treatment _________________________Yes ____ No____

Name of Medication_____________________________________

Time Medication is Taken _______________________________

Possible Side Effects __________________________________

____

____

Likelihood and Frequency of Seizures During School Hours

____

____

Any Limitations Specified by Physician_________________

____

____

Parent's Comments ___________________________________

____

Desired First-Aid Procedures ___________________________

____

____

Signature ___________________________ Date _________

Index